Mind Over Gray Matter:

A New Approach to Dementia Care

Samuel T. Gontkovsky, PsyD

Kathy N. Johnson, PhD, CMC

James H. Johnson, PhD

Lily Sarafan, MS

The information contained in this book is intended to provide helpful and informative material on the subject addressed. It is not intended to serve as a replacement for professional medical advice. Any use of the information in this book is at the reader's discretion. The authors and publisher specifically disclaim any and all liability arising directly or indirectly from the use or application of any information contained in this book. A health care professional should be consulted regarding your specific situation.

ISBN 978-0-9857236-1-3

OTHER BOOKS BY THE AUTHORS

Happy to 102: The Best Kept Secrets to a Long and Happy Life

The Handbook of Live-in Care: A Guide for Caregivers

From Hospital to Home Care: A Step by Step Guide to Providing Care to Patients Post Hospitalization

The Five Senses: A Sensible Guide to Sensory Loss

Comfort Foods Cookbook: A Healthy Twist on Classic Favorites

ACKNOWLEDGMENTS

This book is dedicated to all those who live with dementia, both as patients and as caregivers.

TABLE OF CONTENTS

INTRODUCTION:
BECOMING A DEMENTIA CAREGIVER

Jackie's cognitive decline occurred so slowly that her husband, Michael, scarcely realized that he was becoming a caregiver to a person with dementia. On many days, he was able to convince himself that there was nothing wrong with Jackie—just the usual forgetfulness we all experience when we have a lot on our minds. "She's just a little absent-minded," he told concerned friends and family members. "Who isn't from time to time?"

When Jackie's doctor told Michael that Jackie hadn't scored well on cognitive function tests, Michael brushed off this information as well, responding, "Jackie's always been a little nervous around doctors. She was probably too anxious to concentrate on those tests."

Despite all his efforts to avoid the truth, Michael was finally forced to face his wife's illness on a chilly December evening. He had taken Jackie out for a drive to look at the holiday lights around the neighborhood, an activity she had always enjoyed. On the way home, he stopped by the grocery store to pick up some milk. Jackie decided she would wait in the car.

When Michael came out of the store about 10 minutes later, still humming a holiday tune that had been playing inside, he couldn't believe his eyes. The passenger door of his white Toyota Corolla was open and Jackie was gone. After frantically looking around the parking lot, Michael called the police. With the help of a patrol car, a frantic Michael eventually found Jackie three blocks away from the grocery store. She was weeping in frustration as she tried to open the locked passenger door of a white car that looked similar to Michael's. When the officers approached Jackie, she could not tell them her name. She said she was looking for her mother, even though her mother had passed away more than a decade earlier.

"You can't ever leave her alone like that again," one of the police officers told Michael sternly. "Suppose she had wandered into the middle of a busy street?"

Michael finally acknowledged what he had suppressing for a long time: Jackie was suffering from Alzheimer's disease.

Ellen had known for several months that there was something "off" about her husband Dan's behavior. Always a mild-mannered man, he was becoming more easily agitated—shouting and cursing at even the smallest provocation. He also exhibited unfounded suspicion, convinced that their trusted neighbors of 20 years were stealing his valuables whenever he left home.

One night, when he and Ellen were alone in their house chatting over dinner, Dan started demanding to see his "real wife."

Ellen tried to explain that she was the only wife Dan had ever had.

"You're an imposter!" he yelled at her. "Leave my house now!"

Ellen ran out of the house confused and scared. Trembling, she used her cell phone to call their adult son, Eric. She waited outside the house until he arrived. When the two of them entered the house together, Dan seemed like his normal self again. He had no memory of calling Ellen an imposter or telling her to leave their house. "That would be crazy," he said, but at his wife and son's insistence, he finally agreed to visit his doctor for a check-up.

After weeks of testing, Dan was diagnosed with Pick's disease, a type of dementia that affects the frontal lobe of the brain and can result in hallucinations, paranoia and problems with impulse control.

Like Michael in the previous story, Ellen suddenly found herself in the role of a dementia caregiver.

Having someone you care about diagnosed with Alzheimer's disease, or a related incurable dementia, is a heartbreaking experience. In addition to the stress that comes with watching your loved one's cognitive abilities decline, you must also take on the stress of becoming a principal decision-maker. Will your loved one be able to remain at home? Who will be his or her primary caregiver? How will you handle dangerous issues like driving or wandering? Most importantly, what can you do to ensure that your loved one gets the very best care available?

This book can help you make informed decisions regarding the care of your loved one. We will educate you about the symptoms of dementia, the spectrum of diseases that can cause dementia, state-of-the-art medical and non-medical care options and how to best handle the most common challenges and issues associated with the disease. We'll also inform you about Home Care Assistance's proprietary Balanced Care Method™, a holistic approach to care that promotes healthy longevity and quality of life in typical and atypical aging. We will touch on our exciting new Dementia Therapeutics™ program, which revolves around cognitive interventions specifically designed to delay the onset of dementia symptoms or slow the decline of functioning in people diagnosed with progressive dementias, including Alzheimer's disease. Finally, we will provide you with print and online resources for additional support and information.

Caring for a loved one with Alzheimer's or dementia is not easy, but the information in this book can help make the journey more bearable for you and your loved one.

CHAPTER ONE:
WHAT IS DEMENTIA?

Dementia is sometimes mistakenly believed to be part of the natural aging process. In reality, however, dementia is a cluster of symptoms that manifest as impairments in various cognitive processes, including memory, language, perception, judgment and reasoning.

If your loved one is showing signs of dementia, make an appointment with a neurologist, neuropsychologist or psychiatrist who specializes in the diagnosis and treatment of people with cognitive deficits.

Signs and Symptoms

Memory loss. Memory loss, especially short-term memory loss, is one of the most recognizable signs of dementia. Short-term memory refers to the storage of recently learned information and current events—events that occurred only a few minutes or a few hours before the person is asked to recall them. Even though short-term memory is compromised early on, long-term memory often remains intact until the very last stages of the disease progression. Thus, a person with dementia may not be able to remember that her daughter visited her less than an hour ago, but she may still be able to perfectly describe the birthday party she threw for her daughter 40 years ago.

Trouble with Language. Communication problems can manifest in three primary ways, affecting the ability to produce language, comprehend language or both. A person with dementia may have trouble making sense of the words another person is saying or coming up with the names of familiar people and objects as well as common words. Language problems can be extremely frustrating for both the person with dementia and his or her caregiver.

Problems with Executive Functions. Most of us aren't up for planning a major event, such as a fundraising dinner with 200 guests, but a person with dementia may not even be able to plan and organize simple tasks like preparing a microwave meal or writing out a shopping list. Deficits in reasoning often first become apparent when a loved is faced with an unusual situation that poses a significant safety risk. For instance, it may never occur to a person with dementia whose stove has caught on fire to try to extinguish the flames and get safely out of the burning building. A person with dementia may exhibit poor judgment, making unwise decisions, such as investing his or her life savings in a shady deal or stopping in the middle of an intersection to consult a map if he or she or she becomes lost while driving.

Problems with Motor Functions. People with certain types of dementia, such as vascular dementia (caused by the disruption of blood flow to the brain), may have trouble with balance and coordination. For example, people with dementia related to Parkinson's disease may experience "freezing," or the sudden inability to put one foot in front of the other while walking. Other types of movement problems may also be present. These difficulties occur because the parts of the brain responsible for these movements are damaged from the dementia.

Personality and Mood Changes. As someone develops dementia, you may notice changes in personality and mood. People who have always been pleasant and easy to get along with, for instance, may become cold, harsh and judgmental; a once-trusting person might become fearful or suspicious, believing that loved ones are out to get him or her. As the disease progresses, these changes can become more severe, sometimes resulting in argumentative and even violent behavior. Depression and anxiety also are common among individuals with dementia.

Difficulties with Attention and Concentration. People with dementia may show problems remaining focused and staying on task. They may be unable to pay attention to activities for only brief periods of time and may miss parts of conversations leading to confusion and uncertainty.

Agitation in the Evenings. People with dementia tend to become agitated later in the day, a phenomenon commonly called "sundowning". Associated behaviors can include pacing restlessly, crying, asking to go "home" (even if he or she is home) or repeating anxious gestures, such as rubbing hands together or continually picking up an item and then immediately putting it down.

Hallucinations/Delusions. Hallucinations involve sensations that a person sees, hears, smells, etc. that are not perceived by anyone else. Delusions refer to fixed, bizarre beliefs that a person holds on to despite compelling evidence to the contrary. Some types of dementia, such as Lewy body disease, may result in hallucinations and delusions.

Issues with Personal Hygiene. Many people with dementia find bathing or showering unpleasant or confusing. Others simply forget to bathe themselves or to do laundry on a regular basis. Still others may ignore hygiene as a result of decreased or poor judgment. Sometimes people with dementia become incontinent and will either try to hide or continue to wear the soiled clothes.

Losing Things Repeatedly. Everyone misplaces his or her car keys, briefcase, or purse now and then, but repeatedly losing items can be a sign of cognitive decline. Often people with dementia don't realize that they are the ones misplacing the items and will falsely accuse caregivers or loved ones of stealing from them.

Frequently Missing Appointments. Again, everyone forgets a doctor's visit or a social occasion from time to time, but if your loved one starts missing appointments regularly, this may be a cause for concern.

Disorientation. People with dementia often become confused about time and place—forgetting where they are or losing track of the date and time. For instance, a person who is already at home may repeatedly ask others to "take me home." Disorientation can be especially dangerous if the person wanders away from home and then cannot find his or her way back.

Trouble Understanding Spatial Relationships. People with dementia often have difficulty with depth perception, judging distance and determining color or contrast, which can increase fall risk. Difficulty understanding the spatial relationships between objects may result in things being dropped and broken when a person tries to set them on a table or countertop.

Reversible Causes of Dementia

There are a few cases in which dementia-like symptoms result from another underlying, treatable condition. With treatment, these causes of the dementia symptoms can be stopped or reversed. The most common causes of dementia-like symptoms are detailed below:

Depression. In older adults, depression can lead to memory loss, poor self-care, apathy and withdrawal—all symptoms very similar to those of dementia. Treatment with medication and/or talk therapy can help improve cognitive functioning as well as quality of life. If your loved one is exhibiting signs of both dementia and depression, it's a good idea to have him or her evaluated by a neuropsychologist that specializes in working with older clients.

Medication Side Effects. Some medications, such as benzodiazepines, may cause drowsiness, withdrawal from friends and family members, and hindered decision-making. If your loved one's confusion begins or gets worse immediately after starting a new medication, the new medicine might be the culprit. Check with his or her doctor or pharmacist. It's also a good idea to keep a list of the medications your loved one uses (including vitamins and herbal supplements) and make sure that every doctor he or she sees gets a copy of that list. Also, if feasible, have all prescriptions filled at the same pharmacy. Doing so allows the pharmacist to be on the lookout for medication interactions that the doctor might have missed. Even if you believe that medication is causing your loved one's cognitive decline, do not discontinue use without first speaking to the doctor who prescribed it.

Malnutrition. The brain thrives when adequate nutritional needs are being met. Just as cars need fuel, the human brain requires certain nutrients in order to function at its highest capacity. Some older people don't eat a healthy diet because they don't have the money to buy nutritious foods. Others have stopped cooking, sometimes after the death of a spouse, and eat whatever happens to be on hand, which often includes less nutritious options such as potato chips and candy. Chronic substance abuse can also lead to malnourishment. Ensuring

proper nutrition can ensure brain and overall physical health.
(For more information on a brain-healthy diet, see Chapter Four).

Infections. Some infections, like urinary tract infections (UTIs)
and upper respiratory infections (URIs) can cause an older
person to become forgetful and irritable. If your loved one's
confusion came on abruptly or dementia-like symptoms have
suddenly worsened, a visit to the primary care physician is
necessary to evaluate the situation.

Hydrocephalus. This condition occurs when cerebrospinal fluid
accumulates around the brain, increasing pressure and causing
damage and impairments in cognitive function. Among seniors,
symptoms can include memory loss, poor coordination or
balance, progressive loss of reasoning skills and incontinence
–also symptoms of dementia. A shunt placed to drain away
the excess fluids can relieve pressure on the brain and prevent
further damage from occurring.

Metabolic Dementia. Sometimes disorders of the liver and
pancreas can disturb the balance of chemicals in the blood and
lead to dementia-like symptoms. If these disorders are treated
quickly, the symptoms of dementia can often be reversed. If the
chemical imbalance continues, however, it may start to destroy
brain cells which would cause dementia symptoms to become
permanent.

Wernicke-Korsakoff's Syndrome. Wernicke-Korsakoff's
Syndrome is usually related to years of severe alcohol abuse that
results in a lack of thiamine, also known as vitamin B1. The first
symptoms usually occur as Wernicke's encephalopathy and
involve jerky eye movements, unsteadiness and mild memory loss.

If Wernicke's is not treated immediately, it can develop into Korsakoff's Syndrome, which affects the ability to learn new skills and results in personality changes, hindered decision-making ability, and poor short-term memory. The people affected are usually between the ages of 45 and 65. If treated immediately with thiamine supplements, the cessation of alcohol use and the adoption of a healthy diet, the damage caused by Korsakoff's may be stopped and, in some cases, reversed. Improvement can be seen within two years of initiating therapy. About a quarter of the people affected will make a full recovery, half will make a partial recovery, and the remaining quarter will make no recovery at all.

Irreversible Causes of Dementia

Unfortunately, most types of dementia are degenerative, meaning that they cannot be cured, and progressive, meaning that they get worse over time (see Chapter Two for a discussion of the stages of dementia). Degenerative types of dementia include:

Alzheimer's disease. Alzheimer's disease is the most common type of dementia among people aged 65 and older. It progresses slowly, usually over a period of seven to 10 years, and by the late stages it shuts down almost every brain function. Alzheimer's disease is distinguished by the presence of sticky plaques, made of a substance called amyloid, between the nerve cells of the brain and neurofibrillary tangles, or tangles within the neurons that impede communication input and output.

Vascular dementia. This is the second most common type of dementia and results from disruption of blood flow to the brain. It is often referred to as multi-infarct dementia because it may caused by a series of small strokes, or infarctions. Unlike

Alzheimer's disease, where the decline is slow and steady, a person with vascular dementia sometimes stabilizes for a few weeks and then has a rapid decline if another small stroke occurs. Because disruption of blood flow can affect different parts of the brain, the severity of dementia symptoms and the order in which these symptoms occur will vary from person to person.

Parkinson's disease dementia (PDD). Only about 20% of people with Parkinson's disease develop PDD, usually 10 to 15 years after they are first diagnosed with Parkinson's. Symptoms often include further loss of motor skills and the inability to concentrate, reason and plan.

Lewy body dementia (LBD). Lewy body dementia, a leading cause of dementia in the elderly, occurs when cells start to die in a person's cortex and mid-brain. The remaining cells contain abnormal structures known as Lewy bodies. Lewy bodies can cause symptoms typical of Alzheimer's disease (e.g., memory loss), as well as the loss of motor skills seen in Parkinson's related dementia. People with Lewy body dementia often report vivid hallucinations that are usually not upsetting (e.g., claiming to see a child playing when no one is actually there).

Pick's disease. Pick's disease destroys cells in the temporal and frontal lobes of the brain. Since the frontal lobe is responsible for the regulation of emotions and behaviors, people with Pick's disease often experience personality changes. They may become physically or emotionally abusive or behave inappropriately in public (e.g., laughing at a funeral, urinating in the show room of a store). Unlike most other types of dementias, which tend to largely affect seniors, Pick's disease is most prevalent among people between 40 and 60 years of age.

HIV-related dementia. HIV, or human immunodeficiency virus, is the virus that causes Acquired Immune Deficiency Syndrome (AIDS). When the virus attacks the brain, it causes impaired memory and concentration, apathy, and withdrawal from friends, family and social groups. The newest HIV drugs cannot completely prevent HIV-related dementia, but they can delay its onset for a significant period of time.

Chronic Traumatic Encephalopathy (CTE). CTE is a type of dementia that occurs as a result of several injuries to the head. Aside from a loss of motor function that resembles Parkinson's, the symptoms typically mimic those of Alzheimer's: memory loss, confusion, and the inability to plan or reason. CTE used to be called Pugilistic (i.e. boxing) Syndrome because it most frequently affected professional boxers. In recent years, the National Football League has discovered that football players who have taken numerous hits to the head also exhibit these symptoms.

Huntington's disease. Huntington's disease is a degenerative, genetic condition that is passed down through families. It causes the nerve cells in the brain to break down until the remaining brain cells can no longer sustain life. Huntington's causes a person's mobility and cognition to steadily decline as brain cells die. It can also result in psychiatric symptoms like hallucinations and psychosis. Symptoms similar to dementia include confusion, loss of memory, impaired judgment and personality changes. The majority of people affected by this disease begin to show symptoms in their 40s and 50s, but as the gene is passed down, the defect magnifies and symptoms may begin to appear earlier and earlier in successive generations.

Statistics

According to the Alzheimer's Association, 5.4 million people, two-thirds of whom are women, currently live with Alzheimer's disease and related dementias. Fifteen million Americans provide unpaid care to family and friends with dementia.

The Alzheimer Society of Canada reports that 747,000 (14.9%) of Canadians are living with a cognitive impairment, such as dementia. Although there are no statistics specific to dementia caregivers, one in five people over the age of 45 reports providing care to a person with "long-term health problems."

Being a dementia caregiver is never easy, but having comprehensive, up-to-date information available to help you as you care for your loved one can reduce the burden. The next chapter looks at the stages of dementia and explains changes you can expect to see in your loved one as his or her illness progresses.

CHAPTER TWO:
STAGES OF DEMENTIA

Knowing the basic stages of progressive dementia gives you a way to understand what is happening to your loved one and a shorthand way to describe your loved one's condition to others. It's important to remember, though, that not everyone with dementia will follow these stages perfectly. Your loved one may have some characteristics of early-stage dementia and other characteristics more often seen in middle- or late-stage dementia. Each person is unique, and his or her experience with dementia will be unique, as well.

The Alzheimer's Association and other medical models propose a seven-stage approach to cognitive decline, but these models are generally specific to Alzheimer's disease. Since we are also covering other types of progressive dementia, we have adopted a simplified four-stage approach to cognitive decline that is easier to understand and more inclusive.

Mild Cognitive Impairment (MCI)

A person suffering from MCI, sometimes referred to as mild cognitive decline (MCD), is often aware of memory loss and forgetfulness, challenges with planning and organizing and losing things repeatedly; however, the changes are so slight that even close family and friends may not notice them. Similarly, routine mental status exams and other brief cognitive function tests often do not detect MCI, although it may be diagnosed with a more comprehensive neuropsychological evaluation. MCI generally precedes the onset of early-stage dementia by about seven years.

Experiencing MCI is often frightening for the patient. Some people become angry or depressed. They may stop taking care of themselves and lose the will to live since they realize they are losing control over their mental faculties and know it will only worsen over time.

According to Dr. Sheldon Zinberg, founder of *Nifty after Fifty* (see resources), it is during this stage that medications and changes in lifestyle have their greatest efficacy. Seniors with MCI who stay active display a slower cognitive decline than those who are sedentary. In fact, according to Dr. Zinberg, getting appropriate aerobic exercise and weight-resistance training during this stage of mild cognitive decline can slow the progression of the condition by months or even years.

Early Stage Dementia

Once the person has progressed to early stage dementia, cognitive issues and changes become increasingly clear to friends, family members and the individual's care team. Symptoms begin to interfere with daily activities and hobbies. In addition to short-term memory loss, trouble completing complex tasks and increased confusion, people with early-stage dementia may start to miss appointments, display poor judgment and struggle with reasoning. They tend to "sundown," or have increased trouble with cognitive tasks during the evening hours. You may also begin to see personality and mood changes such as defensiveness or withdrawing from social contact.

As a caregiver, you may also begin to notice instances of confabulation, or the creation of "false memories." When your loved one confabulates, he or she provides inaccurate information —information he or she genuinely believes is true—about a situation. Due to memory deficits, the person will piece together fragmented memories to construct what he or she believes is accurate, or your loved one may try to figure out, logically, what might have happened and claim that as a memory.

Cora was in the early stages of dementia when she fell at an adult day care program and bruised her forehead. When her husband asked her about the bruise that night, Cora said she had been involved in a minor car accident; she described a scenario in detail involving another car hitting her car, causing her to hit her head on the dashboard. It was a perfectly plausible story, except for the fact that Cora hadn't driven in more than six months.

Some caregivers confuse confabulation with lying and then become angry with their loved ones. Confabulation, however, is not about telling a deliberate untruth. It is about a person who has no memory of an event (in the example above, the bruise) trying to use logic and environmental cues to come up with a likely scenario (in this case, a car accident). Rather than embarrassing the person by disagreeing with him or her or trying to prove the person wrong, make a neutral statement like, "Oh, I'm sorry to hear that happened," and change the subject.

During this early stage of dementia, medications and lifestyle changes can still help slow the progression of the disease. Even though the person may not need assistance with activities of daily living (ADLs) such as getting dressed, standing and walking, taking a bath, or using the bathroom, this is a good time to introduce a professional caregiver from a reputable home care agency. The caregiver can make sure that the person is maintaining a healthy diet (see Chapter Four) and can watch for declines in the person's condition about which family members need to know.

People may remain in the early stage of Alzheimer's disease for several years before the condition progresses. The amount of time they can remain in this early stage is often dependent on several factors, including whether or not they remain cognitively, socially and physically active.

Middle Stage Dementia

During the middle stage of dementia, the symptoms persist and worsen. For instance, people with short-term memory loss may now start to lose older memories as well, even forgetting details from their personal histories. It is also during this stage when incontinence and personal hygiene can become a problem. Problems with spatial relationships increasingly become an issue, and the person may occasionally fall as a result. An around-the-clock caregiver often becomes a necessity.

People in the middle stages of dementia may also begin to get confused and disoriented, even in familiar places. Many caregivers have experienced a loved one's pleas to "take me home" when he or she is, in fact, at home. This disorientation can be dangerous for the person who wanders or paces. Sometimes, this person will go out the front door and then not recognize his own house. He or she can wander away looking for a "home" that is actually right in front of him or her.

Other people in middle-stage dementia get lost while driving or get out of their cars and walk away from them. People who wander usually do not recognize potential dangers, such as a busy intersection or an approaching train. In fact, they may be frightened by the light and the sound of oncoming traffic and, without the appropriate cognitive reasoning, simply freeze right in front of an oncoming car.

The person in the middle stage of dementia not only begins to forget familiar places, he or she may also forget familiar people. For example, he or she may ask an adult son or daughter, "Now, how do I know you again?" The patient may also deny knowing a spouse to whom he or she has been married for decades. This can cause a great deal of anguish for family members or other loved ones who feel that they have been forgotten.

Sleep disorders also tend to become a prominent issue in middle-stage dementia. Often your loved one will confuse night and day, or he or she will want to get up at night and wander around. This unsupervised wandering can be dangerous if your loved one lets himself or herself outside or swallows non-food items such as beads or coins.

The person experiencing middle-stage dementia may also begin to have trouble communicating. He or she may talk in "word salad" (a jumble of words that don't make sense strung together) or forget the names of common household items, such as a comb or fork. He or she may also have trouble understanding what loved ones are trying to say to him or her.

Finally, people with middle-stage dementia may undergo more pronounced personality transformations. They may become easily angered or agitated, especially in the later part of the day. They may also develop hallucinations, delusions and compulsions.

Alfred developed the delusion that his wife of 50 years was trying to kill him by putting poison in his food. He refused to eat anything she prepared and began to lose an alarming amount of weight. Alfred's wife finally arranged for a caregiver to prepare all of Alfred's food. As Alfred came to know and trust the caregiver, he began eating again and his health improved.

Many of the medications that have been developed to help people with dementia begin to lose their effectiveness during the middle stage of the disease process. While it is always a good idea for people to eat healthful foods, engage in regular cognitive stimulation and get an adequate amount of exercise, these measures may still slow but will typically no longer reverse the progression of dementia. The middle stage of the disease process usually lasts around four years.

Late Stage Dementia

People in this stage of cognitive decline may lose their ability to communicate verbally beyond short phrases or even one or two words, which they may repeat over and over (for instance, "help me" or "I'm scared"). More commonly, they may not pronounce words correctly or they may speak in confusing sentences, if in sentences at all. They may also experience difficulty understanding language. This makes non-verbal cues an important part of communication.

Oftentimes, they lose muscle control and struggle to smile, swallow, walk, or even sit up without support. The muscles in the arms and legs may become rigid.

They may weep silently or sob at times and may pull away from even the gentlest touch. Their appetite is generally poor, and some weight loss can be expected. Maintaining hydration can be difficult as your loved one's fluids may need to be thickened to make swallowing easier for him or her.

The person is now fully dependent on others to help with almost every facet of his or her life, including basic tasks, including feeding and personal care. He or she is also more prone to injuries and infections such as urinary tract infections, pneumonia, skin tears and bed sores.

Bed sores are often one of the hardest conditions for a caregiver to face. *"I'm doing everything right,"* one spouse exclaimed. *"I'm feeding her, I'm turning her every half hour, and she still looks like no one has been attending to her needs or taking proper care of her."*

The woman's husband needed to hear reassurance that he was doing a good job and that it was his wife's disease process, not any lack of care on his part, that was causing the worsening bedsores and the weight loss.

Although late stage dementia is considered a terminal condition, dementia patients may survive in this state for a few years, depending on how aggressively family members choose to treat the infections and wounds (see Chapter Fifteen).

The next chapter will look at beneficial medications and other treatments recommended for people with dementia.

CHAPTER THREE:
MEDICATION AND OTHER TREATMENTS

Although scientists still hope to uncover a drug therapy that will reverse Alzheimer's symptoms or at least significantly slow their progression, the most recent years of research have been disappointing. In fact, there have been no major changes in drug protocols since the Food and Drug Administration (FDA) approved memantine (Namenda) in October of 2003.

A more promising treatment that has emerged over the past few years is cognitive stimulation and rehabilitation. The focus of cognitive stimulation and rehabilitation is to help keep the brains of people with dementia active. Engaging in cognitive activities can reactivate brain connections that have not been used for some time and can promote new brain connections, which may increasing the functioning of a person with dementia. The ultimate goal of cognitive stimulation is recovering lost cognitive skills and maintaining current skills in order to slow the progression of dementia. Home Care Assistance's exciting new Dementia Therapeutics™ program, which includes cognitive rehabilitation as well as socialization, sensory stimulation, exercise and other scientifically-based interventions, is unique because it focuses on cognitive stimulation and rehabilitation provided to the client within the comfort and safety of the home environment. Until now, treatment of Alzheimer's disease primarily has revolved around medication, and none of the current medications are exceptionally effective.

This chapter will examine the medications that have been approved for the treatment of Alzheimer's disease. For the most part, these medications have not been tested with other forms of dementia. After looking at the medications, we will introduce the concept of cognitive rehabilitation and provide information about Dementia Therapeutics™, available through Home Care Assistance.

Cholinesterase Inhibitors

Cholinesterase inhibitors include donepezil (Aricept), rivastigmine (Exelon) and galantamine (Razadyne). With the exception of Aricept, which is approved by the FDA to treat all levels of the disease process, cholinesterase inhibitors are approved only for the early to middle stages of dementia.

Cholinesterase inhibitors work by temporarily preventing the breakdown of a chemical in the brain called acetylcholine. Acetylcholine is one of the neurotransmitters responsible for carrying messages that are vital for learning and memory through the brain. In theory, higher levels of acetylcholine should improve the communication and functioning of brain cells.

Unfortunately, this is not a one-size-fits-all treatment. According to the Alzheimer's Association, cholinesterase inhibitors are only effective for about half of the people who take them. The people that do benefit from this treatment can expect to see the progression of their disease process slowed for about six months to a year. After that, the medication loses its effectiveness, and cognitive status begins to deteriorate once again.

Side effects may include nausea and vomiting, a decrease in appetite and an increase in bowel movements. In rare cases, the medication makes the person feel so violently ill that he or she decides or is advised by a doctor to discontinue treatment.

Memantine

Memantine, sold as Namenda, is the second type of pharmacological intervention used to treat people with dementia. Its job is to regulate the amount of glutamate in the brain. Glutamate, like acetylcholine, is involved in learning and memory processes. Namenda has been approved by the FDA for use in people who are experiencing middle-stage to severe dementia. Like the cholinesterase inhibitors, Namenda temporarily slows the worsening of dementia symptoms for some people.

The most common side effects of Namenda include headache and constipation, although use of the medication may also result in accelerated heartbeat, chest pain and tightness, coughing and decreased urination. Ironically, using Namenda can also result in confusion and hallucinations for some people with dementia. If your loved one becomes more confused or complains of dizziness or feeling unsteady on his or her feet after starting Namenda, talk to the prescribing doctor right away. Your doctor may want to lower the dose of the Namenda or discontinue the medication altogether.

Some doctors report seeing better results when people with dementia take both Aricept and Namenda.

Vitamin E

As an antioxidant, Vitamin E helps protect brain cells from normal wear and tear as well as from disease processes. More recent studies suggest that high levels may help delay the progression of dementia to more severe stages. People who take these amounts of Vitamin E, however, also have a slightly higher risk of dying from coronary artery disease.

Always talk with your loved one's physician before starting a Vitamin E trial, and follow the physician's recommendations. It is important to note that Vitamin E is not an FDA-approved treatment for mild cognitive impairment or dementia.

Other Medications

At this time, there are no other medications on the market that improve cognitive functioning or delay the dementia disease process. If your loved one is very agitated or aggressive, doctors might prescribe medication to help calm him or her.

Medications typically used in these cases include atypical antipsychotics (e.g., Seroquel, Risperdal) and anti-anxiety medications (e.g., Xanax, Ativan). Your doctor may also suggest a trial of antidepressants if your loved one starts to be withdraw, lose interest in previously enjoyed activities or experience consistent sadness.

Cognitive Intervention and Rehabilitation

Cognitive intervention is a type of treatment developed to help people with cognitive impairments learn new skills, relearn old skills, and maintain the highest level possible of cognitive functioning. Initially developed for people who had suffered an acute cognitive impairment from an event, such as a head injury or a stroke, recent research suggests that cognitive rehabilitation does have clinically significant benefits for people with degenerative impairments including MCI and early-stage dementia.[1]

According to an independent panel convened by the National Institutes of Health, there may be a relationship between cognitive

---

[1] Clare L. 2012. Cognitive rehabilitation and people with dementia. In: JH Stone, M Blouin, editors. International Encyclopedia of Rehabilitation. Available online: http://cirrie.buffalo.edu/encyclopedia/en/article/129/

stimulation and a reduction in cognitive deterioration associated with dementia.

Cognitive rehabilitation is not a one-size-fits-all program. In fact, it must be carefully tailored to meet the individual needs of the person. The first step of cognitive rehabilitation involves an evaluation by a neuropsychologist. This includes assessment of brain functioning across the primary domain of cognition, including attention/concentration, memory, language, visual-spatial perception, and executive functioning. Motor skills are also examined in this process. The neuropsychologist and other members of the professional team meet with the client, family and other relevant parties to discuss the client's history and current symptoms in order to identify personal, realistic and meaningful goals of intervention. A home visit is then scheduled to evaluate the environment in which the client lives in order to make any necessary changes that may increase the client's safety and promote better functioning.

Once the client's particular strengths and weaknesses and various goals have been identified, the neuropsychologist will then prescribe certain exercises, or interventions, to help the client achieve the identified goals, improve functioning and increase quality of life. Interventions may involve:

- Verbal and physical prompts to help the person learn or relearn a daily routine. For instance, the interventionist might prompt an individual not to leave his or her room in an assisted living facility without taking the key. The interventionist might also provide prompts about using equipment (for instance, a CD or a DVD player) or choosing appropriate clothing to start the day.

- Mnemonics or memory activities that help associate one item with another. For instance, your loved one might remember a caregiver's name by thinking, Robin always wears a red uniform.

- Action-based learning. This involves having a person repeat an action many times until it becomes part of his or her daily routine. The interventionist might, for instance, encourage the client to practice getting dressed until the actions come naturally.

- Memory training involves focusing on remembering basic objects. The interventionist might give a client three words to remember and then quiz him or her about the words a few seconds later, a few minutes later and an hour later. Exercises like this may improve memory.

- Fun exercises that promote paying attention. For instance, the interventionist might read a short story and ask the client to clap every time a certain word is read. Or the interventionist and the client might take turns singing different verses of a song.

- Stress management. Stress can negatively affect one's cognitive abilities. Learning how to relax can help improve mood as well as memory.

Dementia Therapeutics™

Home Care Assistance offers a unique in-home program called Dementia Therapeutics™, designed for all stages of cognitive and functional impairment—from MCI to late-stage dementia. Developed from the scientific literature, Dementia Therapeutics™

is an individually based, holistic program that addresses several facets important to overall health and wellbeing for individuals with cognitive deficits and progressive dementia. Different aspects of the program include nutrition, exercise, sensory stimulation, social stimulation, recreation and development of coping skills to help with emotional adjustment. The most unique and important part of the program is cognitive intervention and rehabilitation.

Dementia Therapeutics™ is designed to help people with cognitive impairments maintain or even increase their level of functioning through a structured, uniquely tailored intervention plan. The interventions offered through the program may delay onset of symptoms in specific domains of cognition where symptoms have not developed and slow the progression, or rate of decline, in domains of cognition where symptoms are already present. In addition to helping clients with cognitive deficits function better, the program may offer a sense of hope and purpose to clients and promote increased quality of life.

Based on an extensive literature review of best practices in dementia care and treatment, the program offers various levels of intervention and care based on the client's unique history, strengths and weaknesses, goals and needs. Interventions are provided within the client's home environment by a Certified Dementia Interventionist on a one-to-one basis. When necessary, a caregiver trained in providing personal assistance with basic and instrumental activities of daily living to people with cognitive impairments can be arranged.

For more information about Dementia Therapeutics™ or for an evaluation, call 650-213-8585 or visit www.DementiaTheraputics.com.

CHAPTER FOUR:
ELEMENTS OF A BRAIN HEALTHY DIET

Doctors have known for centuries that the foods we eat can affect both our mental and physical well-being. While the focus has primarily been on the role of nutrition in promoting heart health, in recent years we have seen a shift towards brain health.

A consistently healthy and balanced diet may protect the brain from disorders, such as Alzheimer's disease and related dementias. It may also help to delay the onset of dementia in people with mild cognitive impairment. For those with middle or late stage dementia, food refusal and eating difficulties may be common, so monitoring nutrition is important to maintain overall health. Thus, making healthy food choices is a key part of dementia prevention and care across the spectrum of dementia disorders and stages.

This chapter examines diet as a means of defense against cognitive decline. It also looks at the unique nutritional needs of people with advanced dementia.

Prevention

Given the key role of eating a balanced, healthy diet in disease prevention, before describing the nutritional needs of people who have been diagnosed with dementia, it is important to also review the preventive role of nutrition in cognitive decline. It is common for family caregivers or individuals who are faced with the stress of adapting to the challenges of living with a loved one with dementia to put less focus on attending to their own health, especially nutritional needs. The following tips are useful for all adults in the prevention of cognitive decline:

Manage body weight. According to the Alzheimer's Association, people who are clinically obese at middle age are twice as likely to be diagnosed with dementia in old age as are people with a normal body weight.

Reduce content of high fat foods. One easy way to do this is to select baked or grilled foods instead of fried ones. For an occasional treat, remember that mono- and poly-unsaturated fats, such as those found in olive oil, can actually help raise your levels of HDL (good cholesterol).

Eat brain-protective foods. Foods high in antioxidants, including dark-skinned fruits, colorful vegetables and foods high in omega-3 fatty oils, such as salmon, are considered brain-protective foods. Make sure they have a prominent place in your daily diet.

Cut back on foods high in refined sugar. Refined sugar can cause sharp peaks and drops in your blood glucose level. Over time, these highs and lows may have a damaging effect on the brain.

Stay hydrated. Try to drink approximately half your body weight in ounces of fluid every day. For instance, if you weigh 150 pounds, you should drink at least 75 ounces of water per day. This is between nine and ten eight-ounce glasses of water. (To add variety, you can substitute another unsweetened, non-caffeinated beverage such as herbal tea.)

Dementia Care

Both weight gain and weight loss are common problems as dementia advances. You will need both patience and creativity to address these concerns if they arise.

Weight Gain

Marcia had always had a sweet tooth, but as her Alzheimer's disease progressed, she refused to eat anything but her favorite brand of chocolate ice cream. To make things worse, she often forgot when she had last eaten and accused her husband of "starving" her. Left to her own devices, Marcia would eat two or three cartons of ice cream every day. Such a pattern of behavior resulted in severe weight gain, so much so that it became difficult for her husband to assist her in walking and transferring her from a chair to the bed. In spite of her weight gain, she was also malnourished from consuming so many empty calories.

If your loved one overeats like Marcia, the following tips may help:

Introduce healthy foods along with the person's favorite food. Marcia's husband, for instance, began placing chopped walnuts in her ice cream or topping it off with peanut butter in an effort to get Marcia to eat more protein.

Hide the favorite food. Make it a point to "run out of" your loved one's favorite food a few times a week. When the preferred food is not available, your loved one may be persuaded to eat a healthier alternative.

Serve small portions throughout the day. It's not uncommon for a person with dementia to forget when he or she last ate. Marcia, for instance, insisted she hadn't been fed for days, even if she'd just consumed a meal. Instead of arguing with your loved one, one possible alternative may be to offer small portions of food throughout the day rather than a traditional breakfast, lunch and dinner.

Offer alternative activities. Some people with dementia eat continuously out of boredom or habit. Try suggesting something else you and your loved one could do together like folding the laundry, playing a game of cards, or taking a walk.

Weight Loss

Gerald's problem was exactly the opposite of Marcia's. Food held no interest for him at all. His daughter, who was caring for him at home, could scarcely coax him to take a few bites of food a day and he lost an alarming amount of weight.

There are several possible culprits when dementia patients lose interest in food. They may be taking medication or experiencing brain changes from the disease that alters the smell and taste of familiar foods. If served a large, diverse meal, they may be too overwhelmed by all the choices available. Finally, people experiencing end-stage dementia may forget what food is for or be unable to carry out the motor steps involved in eating due to the disease. They also may develop problems with chewing and swallowing.

If your loved one is refusing food, try these strategies:

Talk to your loved one's doctor. If the problem is related to medication, the doctor may be able to change the dose or prescribe a different medication that doesn't hinder the senses. The doctor may also prescribe an appetite stimulant to help your loved one regain lost weight.

Encourage exercise. Gerald, for instance, spent most of his days dozing in his easy chair. He never did anything to work up an appetite. When his daughter started taking him for a walk around the block before lunch, Gerald's appetite improved and he ate more.

Keep it simple. Heidi Hanna, a PhD in holistic nutrition and author of the books Sharp: Simple Strategies to Boost Brain Power and The Sharp Solution, advises serving a person with advanced dementia only one or two foods at a time. Overstimulation often leads to confusion and agitation.

Make sure the food stands out. Many people with dementia experience problems with vision and depth perception. Thus, a person with dementia might not be able to see a spoonful of mashed potatoes or scrambled eggs against a white plate. Investing in some brightly colored plastic plates can solve this problem.

Try finger foods. Some people with dementia become restless and spend most of their time pacing or wandering. Sitting down to eat feels restrictive, so they may refuse food altogether. Finger foods like small sandwiches, apple slices, celery, or peanut butter on a cracker can be an ideal solution in that your loved one can carry them with him or her and eat them while walking.

Honor preferences. There comes a time in the end stage of dementia when most people lose all interest in food. When that time comes, feed your loved one whatever he will accept. At this end stage, all calories are good calories.

Alter food consistency. People in advanced stages of dementia may not be able to chew or swallow. If your loved one holds food in his or her mouth or chokes on food, notify his doctor. The doctor may suggest pureeing foods and thickening liquids to make them easier to swallow.

Pica

Pica refers to eating inappropriate objects with no nutritional value such as dirt or paper.

When Joan developed advanced dementia, she could no longer distinguish between food and the cups or plates on which it was served. One day, she chipped a tooth while trying to eat a china coffee cup. After a consultation with Joan's doctor, her family started serving all of her meals using paper plates and cups. They also hired a highly trained live-in caregiver to supervise Joan more closely to ensure she consumed nutritious foods regularly. These strategies took care of the problem.

If your loved one suffers from pica, he or she may try to eat anything small enough to fit in his or her mouth. People with dementia-related pica have been known to eat jewelry, pocket change, buttons, houseplants and sometimes even feces. Close supervision, removal of small objects, and storing cleaning supplies and medications in a locked cabinet are the best ways to ensure the safety of your loved one. It may also help to provide a tray of finger foods so that if your loved one gets hungry there is something edible immediately on hand.

The Balanced Care Method™

Based on studies of the extraordinarily long-living elders in the Okinawa region of Japan, Home Care Assistance developed its proprietary approach to care, the Balanced Care Method™. In Okinawa, most people lead long and healthy lives with low, almost nonexistent incidences of disease and cancer. Part of the reason for this incredible longevity is their focus on nutrition;

the typical diet in the Okinawa region consists of vegetables, fruits, whole grains, lean proteins and omega-3 fatty acids. Likewise, all Home Care Assistance caregivers trained in the Balanced Care Method™ are taught to focus on healthy nutrition for their clients.

In fact, Home Care Assistance is the only home care agency that provides culinary training for caregivers. The company has partnered with trained chefs to teach caregivers basic meal preparation and nutrition to improve their culinary skills and ultimately improve the quality of the meals they serve their clients.

To complement Home Care Assistance's philosophy of healthy longevity, the company even combined their favorite Balanced Care Method™ friendly recipes into their *Comfort Food Cookbook* so that caregivers and clients could access them easily.

CHAPTER FIVE:
DEMENTIA AND LEGAL CONCERNS

With an increase in diagnosed cases, people are more aware of dementia and its symptoms now than ever before. With so much focus on biological and psychological studies, doctors are better able to diagnose the disease and intervene before the symptoms become debilitating. An early diagnosis not only increases a person's chance of delaying cognitive decline, but it also gives people an opportunity to get their legal affairs in order while their mental faculties are still intact.

If your loved one has been diagnosed with mild cognitive impairment or early stage dementia, he or she should consider preparing the following documents:

Living Will

A living will is a document that tells your doctor and your family what kind of treatment you want at the end of your life. For instance, you can specify whether you would accept or refuse chemotherapy, surgery, IV fluids or feeding tubes. Completing a living will is a courtesy to your loved ones because it removes the burden of their having to guess what kind of treatments you would or would not accept.

Two conditions generally must be met in order for a living will to go into effect. First, you must be unable to make decisions (incapacitated) or to speak for yourself. Second, two doctors must certify that you have a terminal condition and will die soon, or that you will never regain a quality of life that is acceptable to you. You can obtain a living will form from your local hospital.

An elder and disability law attorney can also draw up a living will for you. Be aware that some states require the signature of a notary for the document to be valid; others only require the signature of one or two witnesses who are not related to you. Verify your state laws before completing the document.

Durable Power of Attorney for Healthcare

A durable power of attorney (DPOA) for healthcare is a document that allows individuals to name a person, called an agent, who can make healthcare decisions on their behalf when they are no longer able to make decisions for themselves.

Typically, a DPOA for healthcare grants the agent the right to accept or refuse treatment on an individual's behalf, to hire or discharge healthcare workers and to transfer an individual to a skilled nursing facility, or other institution, if safety becomes an issue.

The document is called a durable power of attorney because it endures even after an individual become incapacitated. A regular power of attorney terminates once a person loses the ability to make decisions for himself or herself.

Almost anyone over the age of 18 years can serve as the DPOA agent to whom responsibilities are entrusted. The most common choices include a spouse or partner, an adult child, or a close friend. Alternate agents can also be named in the event that the first choice is unavailable or unwilling to take on the responsibility.

There is flexibility in deciding whether the DPOA for healthcare will go into effect immediately, or whether it will commence only when one or two doctors certify that the person is incapacitated and can no longer make reasonable decisions.

DPOA for healthcare forms are available at most local hospitals. An elder and disability law attorney can also draw up a DPOA. As with the living will, check your state's laws to find out whether this document requires the signature of a notary.

Outside the Hospital Do Not Resuscitate

A "Do Not Resuscitate" (DNR) form is a medical order signed by both the individual and a physician. The form tells paramedics and other healthcare workers that if a person's heart stops beating or if his or her breathing stops, resuscitative attempts should not be made. (In other words, the person does not want to receive rescue breathing, chest compressions, or electric shocks in an attempt to restart the heart.)

In the absence of this form, an individual is considered a "full code," and healthcare workers will do everything they can to restore life, even if an individual is very ill and his or her quality of life is poor.

Some people are put off or confused by the term "do not resuscitate." For this reason, some states have renamed the form "Allow Natural Death," or AND.

A DNR or AND form is available at your local hospital. You can also obtain one from the company that provides emergency medical services in your community (Note: To be valid, a DNR or AND must be co-signed by a physician).

Durable Power of Attorney for Finances

A DPOA for finances allows an individual to name an agent who can take care of financial matters when an individual is no longer deemed able to handle them.

Although there are do-it-yourself forms online or kits available at some office supply stores, it is better to have an attorney draw up a DPOA for finances. Any attorney can create these documents, but attorneys that specialize in elder and disability law usually have the most experience.

Make sure that the document specifies that this is a *durable* power of attorney. As discussed before, a regular power of attorney terminates when an individual become unable to make decisions for himself or herself, so it is less useful in cases when the person has Alzheimer's disease or dementia.

It is also important to make sure that the DPOA for finances gives your agent the right to apply for public benefits such as Medicaid, the right to make gifts on your behalf, and the power to add assets to or remove them from any trust you may have.

When designating an agent to make financial decisions for you, choose someone whom you trust completely and talk to that person to make sure he or she is aware of your wishes. If you don't have anyone that you trust with your money, you can designate your lawyer to be your agent for financial decisions. You can also designate two agents and stipulate that they both have to agree before any financial decisions can be carried out on your behalf.

Will

A will is a legal document that specifies what will happen to an individual's assets when he or she dies. A will can also be used to appoint a guardian for any minor children under your care.

Again, although do-it-yourself kits are available, it is wiser to have a will drawn up by an attorney. This is especially true in cases where there may be disagreement or someone may contest the will. An attorney can help plan for different scenarios and make sure that everything in the will complies with applicable laws and regulations. Some states, for instance, require that you leave a certain percentage of your assets to your spouse.

Canada Laws

If you live in Canada, the laws may be slightly different than they are in the United States. Additionally, each of the provinces has a slightly different set of rules and requirements. In Saskatchewan, for instance, you can complete a health care directive if you are 16 years of age or older. In Alberta, you must be over 18 years old, and the form is called a personal directive. British Columbia has a Representation Agreement Act which requires that all agreements be registered with the registrar before going into effect. For further information and assistance with legal planning, contact the Canadian Centre for Elder Law (**http://www.bcli.org/ccel; 604-822-0633**) or visit the CBC News site for frequently asked questions about end of life planning: **http://www.cbc.ca/news/background/wills/**.

CHAPTER SIX:
MEDICAL AND DENTAL CARE

Managing the issues and needs of a loved one with dementia is stressful and taxing. When a loved one has additional health-related problems, care becomes even more complex and demanding. Here we will discuss the most common medical problems that co-exist with dementia, the complications that occur with them, and care options, namely curative and palliative care. We also address the importance of routine medical and dental care in preventing serious health problems.

Infections

Seniors are especially vulnerable to urinary tract infections (UTIs) and upper respiratory infections (URIs). In addition, as dementia progresses and your loved one begins to have trouble chewing and swallowing, he or she may actually inhale food into the lungs, a process called aspiration. When food is inhaled into the lungs, the lungs recognize it as an irritant and as a foreign body and signal the immune system accordingly. This leads to swelling, inflammation and often pneumonia.

Typically, the initial signs of a UTI are burning or itching during urination and cloudy urine. In seniors with dementia, however, the first signs of infection manifest as increased confusion and irritability. Thus, if your loved one exhibits sudden changes in mood and cognitive status, you should notify the primary doctor to check for the presence of a UTI. If the doctor does determine your loved one has a UTI, he or she can order a culture to assess which antibiotics would be most successful in treatment. Once the infection is gone, your loved one will usually return to his or her normal level of functioning.

A URI, such as the common cold or bronchitis, is usually diagnosed when your loved one develops a persistent cough, nasal congestions and sore throat. A URI can be caused by bacteria, which can be treated with antibiotics, or more commonly a virus, in which case treatment consists only of alleviating the symptoms. Some doctors will also want your loved one to have a chest X-ray to be sure that he or she does not have pneumonia. Most doctors will try an initial round of antibiotics to see if your loved one's condition improves. In any case, the infection will usually run its course in seven to ten days. Recovery from a URI is difficult to predict, depending on additional complications that may arise. Many people return to their previous level of functioning, but others are weakened by the ordeal and their health declines noticeably.

Lung Disease

Lung disease, also called chronic obstructive pulmonary disease, COPD, or emphysema, is most common in smokers and in people who have been exposed to pollutants over a long period of time. Like dementia, it is a progressive disease, meaning it gets worse as time goes on. Certain medical treatments and lifestyle changes, however, can slow the progression and give your loved one more years of relatively good health.

When COPD is diagnosed, most doctors recommend that the patient stop smoking immediately, if applicable. If your loved one with dementia still smokes, talk to the doctor about a nicotine patch to lessen withdrawal symptoms. Then unobtrusively remove all of the cigarette packs from the house. Your loved one may not even remember smoking, especially if he or she is not craving nicotine. Some people, however, miss having a cigarette in their mouth. If that is the case, try giving your loved one an unlit or electronic cigarette, used to simulate the act of tobacco smoking, and see if that satisfies him or her. If your loved one still insists on smoking, explain in simple terms that his her lungs are sick and will get worse if the smoking continues.

Inhaled medications, delivered by an inhaler or a nebulizer, are generally used to control COPD in its initial stages. Your loved one puts the mouthpiece into his or her mouth and inhales deeply, drawing the medication into the lungs. In the middle to later stages of dementia, some people are no longer able to use a mouthpiece effectively. If this is true for your loved one, you may consider getting a clear mask that covers the mouth and nose, allowing him or her to breathe normally to get the most benefit out of the treatment.

A final treatment for lung disease is supplemental oxygen. This is usually delivered by a nasal cannula, or two prongs that fit just inside of the nostrils. Depending on the condition of your loved one's lungs, your doctor may suggest he or she use the oxygen only at night, only when engaging in physical activity such as walking or all of the time. As dementia progresses, the presence of the nasal cannula can increase feelings of confusion and restraint. As with the inhaled treatments, you can try a mask, but this, too, may feel constrictive. Again, you can offer a simple explanation to your loved one that his or her lungs are sick and that the oxygen will help him or her breathe better. Some people dislike the oxygen so much that they simply refuse to wear it. If your loved one does this, notify the physician who prescribed it.

If your loved one requires supplemental oxygen, it is absolutely imperative that you prevent him or her from smoking while the oxygen tank is nearby. Oxygen is flammable; your loved one can get severe burns or set fire to the home. Rather than fight about this issue, tell your loved one that if he or she wants to smoke, he or she must notify you so that you can remove the mask or cannula and move the oxygen concentrator (the device that manufactures the oxygen) into another room. If your loved one forgets to call you, take charge of the cigarettes and only provide them when you are sure there is no fire hazard.

Heart Failure

Congestive heart failure, or CHF, occurs when the heart is unable to pump sufficient amounts of blood, and thus oxygen and nutrients, to meet the body's needs. As a result, the chambers of the heart expand to hold more blood or become thick and stiff in an attempt to increase pumping power. Although this initially keeps the blood flowing, it eventually results in further weakness to the heart and hinders pumping ability. When the pumping ability of the heart declines, the kidneys become damaged and fluid accumulates in the lungs, liver, arms, legs and gastrointestinal tract.

Heart failure can be caused by coronary artery disease, a condition that occurs when the arteries become blocked. It can also be caused by a heart attack that leaves the heart muscle damaged, cardiomyopathy, or damage that is not caused by artery problems, and conditions that place too much strain on the heart such as thyroid or kidney disease.

In the early stages of CHF, the doctor will probably recommend various lifestyle changes including smoking cessation, regular physical activity and a low sodium diet. The doctor will probably also prescribe medications to treat high blood pressure and cholesterol, as these conditions are often the underlying culprits of heart failure. He or she may also prescribe medications to prevent the heart failure from getting worse by strengthening the heart muscle to improve pumping capacity, keeping the blood from clotting and ridding the body of excess fluid and salt.

Some of the medications your loved one may take include angiotensin converting enzyme (ACE) inhibitors that treat both high blood pressure and weak heart muscles, angiotensin II receptor blockers (ARB) that treat coronary artery disease, and beta blockers that are used to treat high blood pressure or people who have had a recent heart attack.

A doctor may recommend surgeries and devices for certain patients. Coronary bypass surgery (CABG) or angioplasty can help improve blood flow while heart valve surgery may be the best option if damaged heart valves are causing the heart failure. A doctor may also suggest implanting a pacemaker or defibrillator to regulate heart contractions and rhythms. He or she may also prescribe supplementary oxygen (see Lung Disease, above).

When treated properly, your loved one with heart failure should be able to participate in almost any activity he or she enjoys including physical exercise. Always talk to your loved one's doctor before undertaking a new activity or exercise program.

Diabetes

Type 1 diabetes is typically diagnosed in children and young adults, and occurs when the body simply stops manufacturing insulin, a substance that converts glucose, or sugar, into a usable form of energy to power our bodies. Type 2 diabetes, on the other hand, is more often diagnosed in adults and occurs when the body, namely the liver and muscle cells, does not respond correctly to insulin. Because glucose cannot enter the cells, high levels build up in the bloodstream, a condition called hyperglycemia. If unchecked, this state can cause damage to the kidneys, the eyes and the nervous system.

If your loved one is diagnosed with Type 2 diabetes, the doctor will probably recommend that he or she cut back on starchy carbohydrates and refined sugar in favor of lean proteins, fruits and vegetables. This can be a challenge for the person with dementia, many of whom have a sweet tooth. If your loved one objects to the changes in his or her diet, speak with the doctor, a nutritionist, or a dietitian, to learn effective strategies to overcome his or her objections. They may suggest giving your loved one small portions of the food he or she enjoys. Alternatively, you can substitute refined sugar with natural sweeteners such as honey and agave, in line with the Balanced Care Method™.

Your doctor will probably also want you to measure your loved one's blood-glucose levels regularly. This is done by lightly pricking the finger or the forearm to get a drop of blood, placing the blood on a test strip, and using a device called a blood-glucose meter, or a glucometer, to check the level of glucose in the blood. Your doctor will tell you how to interpret the numbers. If you handle this process in a calm, matter-of-fact manner, your loved one is more likely to stay calm, as well.

The doctor may also prescribe oral medications or injections of insulin to treat your loved one's diabetes. The injections are given with a small, very sharp needle. Most people don't even feel the shot. Again, if you are calm throughout the process, your loved one probably will be, too.

Cancer

Cancer refers to the unregulated growth of abnormal, or malignant, cells in the body. The uncontrolled dividing cells form tumors and may spread to other parts of the body. Almost any site in the body is vulnerable to cancer and people of any age can be affected, though risk generally increases with age. Because few if any symptoms appear other than a growing mass, cancer is usually diagnosed with a surgical procedure called a biopsy, in which the surgeon removes the tumor and sends a tissue sample to a lab where it is studied under a microscope. The lab reports whether the tumor is benign (harmless) or malignant (cancerous). The patient's treatment team also "stages" the cancer by establishing what kind of cancer is involved and whether or not it has spread to other places in the body.

Typically, a Stage I tumor is confined to the part of the body where doctors first found it, while a Stage IV tumor has spread (metastasized) to different parts of the body (for instance, from the pancreas to the liver). The overall chance of survival varies greatly by location, type and the stage of the tumor when detected.

There are several treatments for cancer including surgery, chemotherapy (medicine taken by mouth, shot, or IV) and radiation. Some cancers grow very slowly, and instead of treatment, your loved one's doctor might suggest close monitoring. That means your loved one will see the doctor at set intervals to run tests. If the cancer becomes more aggressive, treatment is always an option.

Physical Disabilities

Your loved one may require assistance with balance and mobility either due to orthopedic surgery, a fracture or bone break, or a medical condition such as a stroke or Parkinson's disease. If your loved one has difficulty with balance, coordination and mobility that interferes with the completion of routine tasks like walking and feeding, consider hiring a caregiver to monitor his or her safety and comfort. Your loved one's doctor may also recommend rehabilitation services.

A rehabilitation team consists of several members. A physical therapist helps with tasks like walking and getting back and forth between two places like a wheelchair and a bed. An occupational therapist helps with fine motor movements like buttoning a blouse or managing a spoon or fork. An occupational therapist can also provide limited cognitive rehabilitation. A speech therapist helps with chewing, swallowing and speech.

The rehabilitation team will do its best to get your loved one back to the level at which he or she was functioning before the illness or injury. If complete recovery isn't possible, the team may recommend that your loved one use an assistive device like a wheelchair, walker, or cane to make getting around easier.

Problems with Teeth and Gums

People with dementia often forget or lose the ability to brush their teeth because of the disease, which can result in cavities, broken teeth, infections of the gums and sores in the mouth.

Make sure oral care is an important part of your loved one's morning and nighttime routines. If your loved one is unable to brush his or her own teeth, you may have to help by putting toothpaste on the brush, giving him or her verbal cues, or brushing his or her teeth yourself.

When you take over a chore like tooth-brushing or any other type of personal care, be gentle. Do not make a joke about your loved one needing help, even if you are just trying to ease the tension. In fact, once you have provided the care, don't mention it again. This protects your loved one's dignity. If problems with the teeth, gums, or mouth do develop, take your loved one to see a dentist.

Pain

As stated previously, people with dementia often have difficulty communicating. As a result, your loved one may not be able to tell you that he or she is feeling pain or where the pain is located on his or her body. Pain can have multiple causes, including migraine headaches, infections, cavities, arthritis and injuries.

Watch for symptoms of pain like grimacing, crying, yelling out with movement, rubbing the same spot over and over, or "guarding" an area—taking extra care to see that it is not touched. If you suspect your loved one is in pain, you may have to play detective to find out exactly where the pain is located. You should also address your concerns with your loved one's doctor. The doctor may prescribe a mild pain reliever or suggest that your loved one take over-the-counter medication like Tylenol or Aleve.

When Jenny took over her Aunt Sarah's care, she noticed that Sarah often cried and rubbed her right knee. Jenny knew that Sarah had a history of arthritis, so she spoke to Sarah's doctor. The doctor recommended giving Sarah Tylenol twice a day and using an arthritis cream on her knee. Sarah's tears disappeared almost immediately, and her mood improved over the next several weeks. By recognizing her aunt's pain symptoms, Jenny dramatically improved Sarah's quality of life.

Doctor Appointments

Even if your loved one seems to be enjoying good physical health, he or she should still see a primary care physician, the doctor in charge of his or her care, for an annual checkup. It is also important to schedule appointments for flu and pneumonia vaccines. Most doctors suggest that their older patients get these shots regularly. Getting a person with dementia to the doctor's office can be a bit of a challenge, especially if your loved one associates seeing the doctor with getting shots or with other unpleasant treatments.

In some cases, you may be better off not telling your loved one about the doctor's appointment in advance. If you do, he or she may only worry repeatedly about it until the whole idea becomes even scarier than it was already. Instead, wait until the day of the appointment when you and your loved one are in the car and say in a casual tone, "We have some errands today. We need to stop at the grocery store and the library, and we have an appointment to see Dr. Becker."

You can also make things easier on yourself and your loved one by telling the doctor's office staff in advance about your loved one's cognitive problems. Try to get the first appointment of the day so you won't have to wait.

Dental Checkups

An annual dental checkup is a good idea so that the dentist can spot problems early on and address them quickly. As with routine doctor's appointments, don't necessarily tell your loved one about a dental appointment in advance, but do notify the office staff that your loved one has dementia.

Because some people with cognitive problems refuse to open their mouths or try to bite the dentist, your dentist may prescribe a mild oral sedative for your loved one to take prior to the appointment. Depending on the level of anxiety—many older people have had bad experiences with dentists or simply have not made routine dental care a part of their lives—the dentist also might ask you to consider IV sedation at the time of the appointment.

Curative versus Palliative Care

Curative care, sometimes referred to as aggressive care, is any treatment intended to treat or cure a disease. Palliative care, also known as comfort care, is intended to relieve symptoms such as pain, nausea, or anxiety. It is not intended to treat the underlying condition.

Choosing Palliative Care

Doctors usually recommend palliative care when curative care has failed to stop or reverse the disease process. Other instances where you might want to consider comfort care over aggressive treatment include:

When your loved one has made specifications regarding care. If your loved one is able to participate in decision making, if you talked to your loved one about his or her wishes regarding curative versus palliative care, or if he or she executed a living will, do your best to follow your loved one's preferences.

When quality of life may be compromised. Take an honest look at your loved one's quality of life and ask yourself if he or she is content with his current circumstances. If not, focusing on comfort care instead of life-prolonging treatments might be the optimal choice.

When a doctor offers medically-based advice. Ask your doctor about both the benefits and the side-effects you can expect from curative treatment and weigh both carefully. If a treatment has many unpleasant side effects and only a small success rate, it may be time to consider palliative care.

As you manage the physical care of your loved one with dementia, you will also have to address his or her mental health needs. The next chapter examines mental health issues that are common in people with dementia and offers suggestions for managing them.

CHAPTER SEVEN:
MENTAL HEALTH

Nell had survived the Holocaust in Germany, hidden by two of her parents' closest friends. Now in her 80s and suffering from dementia, she no longer recognized her eldest son who had taken responsibility for her care. In fact, she thought he was a member of the Gestapo coming to take her away to a concentration camp.

Sadly, Nell's situation is not unusual. Many people with dementia develop psychological problems including depression, anxiety, hallucinations and paranoid delusions. This chapter will provide some tips on caring for your loved one's mental health.

Depression

Depression Symptoms. Depression in a person with dementia may initially manifest in several ways, some typical for the general population and some not. Your loved one may withdraw from family and friends or lose interest in activities he or she used to enjoy. He or she may also seem angry or irritable most of the time. Another potential symptom of depression is persistent talk of death or suicide, either indirectly ("You'd all be better off if I just died") or directly ("One of these days I'm just going to kill myself"). When people with dementia become depressed, they often spiral into a steep cognitive decline. If the depression is treated successfully, some of that decline may be reversible.

Depression in people with dementia seems to have at least two underlying triggers. People may become depressed as a result of noticing their declining cognitive abilities and independence. This type of depression frequently occurs in people with MCI and early-stage dementia. Treatment will vary on an individual basis. In addition to pharmacological interventions other treatments may include:

Support groups. Many communities offer support groups for people in the early stages of dementia. Participants often find comfort in meeting other people who share their feelings and in exchanging fears, concerns and coping strategies.

Cognitive rehabilitation. Going through cognitive rehabilitation can help your loved one regain some skills and delay losing others. Talk to your doctor or call the local chapter of the Alzheimer's Association to find out where cognitive rehabilitation is available in your community.

Exercise. Exercise releases endorphins that can elevate mood and even improve cognitive function. Encourage your loved one to walk, participate in yoga or water aerobics, or engage in any other kind of physical activity he enjoys.

As noted previously, the new Dementia Therapeutics™ program of Home Care Assistance includes both cognitive rehabilitation and exercise as part of each client's individually-tailored intervention plan.

Be kind and patient. Being a caregiver can be a tough job. There will be days when smiling is the last thing you feel like doing. Your loved one, though, may be more in tune with your moods than you suspect. If you seem down or stressed out, he or she may become upset, as well. If your mood is calm and upbeat, your loved one will reflect that mood, too.

Depression may also be attributed, in part, to brain damage caused by dementia. This type is most common in those with vascular dementia and those in which the subcortical region of the brain has been damaged.

Talk to your doctor about your loved one's depression. He or she will probably suggest a trial of antidepressant medication. Don't be discouraged if the first few medications you try don't seem to help much. No two individuals have exactly the same brain chemistry, and it might take several tries to find the medicine that works best for your loved one.

Depression and Suicide

In the United States, the group most at risk for committing suicide is men over the age of 65 years. In addition, the elderly are more likely to have fatal attempts than youth. In Canada, it is men over the age of 80 years. The greatest risk factors in both countries include having a physical and/or mental illness, isolation, and access to a means with which to end one's life, particularly firearms.

Many people want to silence a loved one who speaks of death or suicide, or brush his or her statements off as "silly". It's better, however, to encourage your loved one to talk about his or her feelings. Don't be afraid that you will somehow give your loved one the idea of committing suicide—he or she has already thought of it, probably many times.

As you talk to your loved one, ask yourself whether he or she has a plan and a means to follow through with it. In general, people who do not have a specific plan ("I just want to go to bed and never wake up") are at a lower risk than people who do

("I'm going to go to your mother's grave and shoot myself with the gun in my bed stand").

If your loved one mentions suicide or keeps bringing up the topic of death, inform his or her doctor or psychiatrist immediately. If you believe your loved one is at immediate risk of harming himself or herself, call 911 at once and request that your loved one be taken to an emergency room for a psychiatric evaluation.

As dementia progresses, the risk of suicide declines; most people in the middle to late stages of the disease process are not able to make a complicated plan and carry it out, although they may attempt self-harm impulsively if a weapon or other means is left within their reach. If your loved one has a history of suicidal thoughts or behavior, make sure to keep his or her living environment safe and free of objects that could potentially cause harm.

Feelings of Anxiety

Your loved one may express feelings of anxiety by crying, pacing, wringing his or her hands, repeatedly looking for lost objects, or crying out repetitively ("Help me!" or "I'm scared!").

Several factors can increase your loved one's feelings of anxiety. One of the chief culprits is a change in your loved one's living environment. This can be a big change, such as moving from him or her home to a skilled nursing facility, or it can be a smaller change, such as moving the furniture in your loved one's room to accommodate a wheelchair or walker. Sometimes, anxiety is the result of the general confusion due to the disease. Your loved one may be looking for his or her childhood home, for example, and not the one they have been living in for the past

15 years. Your loved one may not even recognize you or the place where he or she is currently living.

Fear, often of things that happened in the past, is another common cause of anxiety. Nell, introduced at the beginning of the chapter, kept remembering a time when her life was in danger.

Fatigue can also cause anxiety. If your loved one isn't sleeping well, or has his or her days and nights mixed up, it's possible he or she may be more anxious than usual.

If your loved one with dementia suffers from anxiety, there are many ways you can help. First, keep a log to determine if there are times of day or certain circumstances that seem to make the anxiety worse or better. Nell's son, for example, found that Nell's anxiety got worse in the evening when he was trying to help her get ready for bed. He hired a female caregiver to assist Nell in the evenings, and much of her anxiety vanished immediately.

Always offer reassurance. You might say something like, "It's okay. I'm here to keep you safe. I won't let anything hurt you." You may need to repeat this calming message several times before your loved one understands it and believes it.

If your loved one is ruminating, or thinking about the same upsetting thing over and over, try to redirect his or her attention to something else like eating a snack, helping you fold laundry, or watching a favorite television program.

People with dementia who are anxious tend to have a lot of excess energy, so it may help to take a walk with your loved one, or encourage him or her to spend a few minutes exercising on a treadmill or pedaling a stationary bike if medically cleared to do so.

Your loved one's anxiety may make you anxious as well, but you will be in a better position to soothe your loved one if you try to remain calm. If you feel like you're about to lose your patience, try counting to ten or step outside for a few minutes. The more upset you are, the more upset your loved one is likely to be.

High levels of generalized anxiety, a syndrome marked by patterns of worry, physical tension, difficulty concentrating, irritability, and restlessness, can cause damage to the body, including increased blood pressure, aches and pains, sleep problems, loss of appetite, digestive problems, teeth grinding and clinical depression. Thus, if your loved one's anxiety continues or gets worse in spite of your best efforts, it's time to have a talk with his or her doctor. The doctor may prescribe a low dose of medicine to help your loved one feel calm and relaxed. The most common medications used for this purpose are called benzodiazepines. Some of the brand names you may be familiar with are Ativan, Xanax and Valium. Doctors usually try to avoid prescribing these medications for older patients because side effects include dizziness, drowsiness, and an increased risk of falling. It may be better to risk these side effects, though, if the reduction in anxiety-related symptoms will greatly improve quality of life.

Hallucinations

Hallucinations involve seeing, hearing, or more rarely, smelling something not real and that others do not sense. Hallucinations are common in certain types of dementia, such as Lewy body dementia. They may also be caused by delirium due to medication interactions or infections.

Because of vision problems characteristic of aging and dementia, your loved one may sometimes mistake people on the television for people present in the room, or mistake their own reflection for another person. These are not hallucinations but rather illusions. A hallucination is a false sensory perception unrelated to anything real. An illusion is a misrepresentation or misinterpretation of something real.

The content of hallucinations will vary from case to case. For instance, reports about seeing visions of heaven, angels, or important people who have already died are common in the last days or hours of life.

When David's dementia progressed to middle stage, he began talking to an individual he referred to as his friend, just as if there were another person in the room with him. This didn't bother him in the least. In fact, he seemed to enjoy the company. David seemingly both saw and heard things that weren't actually present. With some misgivings, his family allowed the conversations to continue uninterrupted. They lasted about three months until David lost interest. After that, he never mentioned his "friend" again.

If your loved one is frightened or irritated by the hallucinations, your approach should be somewhat different than the hands-off approach chosen by David's family. First of all, stay calm. Don't try to argue with your loved one or challenge his or her reality ("For heaven's sake, Mom, there's nothing there!"). It's better to say something like, "I don't see it, but I believe you do and I could imagine that would be a bit scary."

Again, it is important to distinguish between hallucinations and illusions. Look for possible sources of the illusions. A chair with a blanket or clothing thrown over it can look like another person or even a ghost to a person with dementia or visual disturbances. You may need to remove mirrors and television sets from your loved one's room. Also, look at the decorations your loved one keeps. Could he or she be confusing a stuffed dog with a real dog or a doll with a living child?

Provide reassurance ("I won't let anything hurt you") and try to redirect your loved one's attention ("Never mind about the little girl now. Her mom will take care of her. Come help me get dinner ready.").

Often, the hallucinations will go away just as quickly as they came. When they continue to occur, however, and when they are upsetting to your loved one, talk to your loved one's doctor. He or she may suggest that your loved one try a class of medications known as atypical antipsychotics. While these medications have not been approved by the FDA to treat hallucinations in dementia patients, they sometimes help. Side effects can include dizziness, tiredness and weight gain. Among elderly patients, atypical antipsychotics may also increase the risk of having a stroke.

Paranoia/Delusions

Paranoia means suspecting others are out to get you when there is no evidence that this is so. Delusions are fixed, untrue beliefs. Nell, who believed that her son was actually a member of the Gestapo coming to arrest her, suffered from paranoid delusions, a combination of the two. Other dementia patients may also develop hurtful delusions about family members or caregivers. Some of the more common delusions include:

- She's stealing my money.
- He's keeping me a prisoner against my will.
- She hurts me.
- He doesn't feed me.

Being accused of abuse or neglect when you're bending over backwards to help your loved one can be devastating. It's even harder if some family members believe what your loved one is saying. Even so, try not to respond with anger or take offense when your loved one says these things. Resist the temptation to try to talk your loved one out of his beliefs. By definition, delusions do not fade in the face of logic.

If the problem can be easily fixed, take care of it. "Here's your brown purse, Mom. It was on the other side of your chair." "I'm sorry you feel like you're starving, Dad. I'll get you something to eat."

If the problem cannot be fixed—for instance, if your loved one is demanding access to talk with the President about an alien invasion—try to redirect him or her to a different topic. "The President is out of the country right now, Dad. Let's play a game of cards."

If your loved one can't be redirected, try stepping out of the room for 15 to 20 minutes—assuming it is safe to leave your loved one alone, of course—and coming back in as if the accusations had never taken place. Chances are your loved one will be focused on something else by the time you return.

When your loved one makes accusations against you, especially when he or she accuses you of stealing money or property, it's a good idea for you to keep careful records of how your loved one's assets are being used. Good record keeping helps cover you in case another family member believes what your loved one is saying.

Psychiatric Hospitalization

George stood over six feet tall and weighed 200 pounds. His wife, Emma, was 5'2" and weighed less than 100 pounds. George had always been a gentle and caring spouse, but as his dementia worsened, he became fixated on the idea that Emma was having an affair. One night he became so agitated, he threw a glass at Emma. She quickly ducked out of the way and the glass shattered against the wall. Emma ran to the home of a neighbor who called the police.

When Emma explained that George had dementia, the police took him to a local emergency room. From there, George was admitted to a gero-psych unit (a psychiatric unit specializing in mental health issues that affect the elderly).

Over the next two weeks, the staff worked to control his delusions and episodes of rage with medications. George was able to come back to his home with the help of a full-time caregiver. He sometimes still talked about Emma having an affair, but he never reacted violently towards her again.

There are times when psychiatric hospitalization may be necessary for your loved one. You should certainly consider it if he or she is violent or actively suicidal.

That said, there are a few drawbacks to psychiatric hospitalization. The sudden change in environment can increase your loved one's confusion. Additionally, if your loved one associates you with the hospitalization, he or she may come to resent you. The resentment itself may last long after the memory of what caused it fades away.

One of the biggest contributors to psychological and emotional wellbeing is a feeling of independence. The next chapter discusses balancing your loved one's progressive dementia with his or her need to manage his or her own life.

CHAPTER EIGHT:
BALANCING DEMENTIA
AND INDEPENDENCE

Most people value their independence and would much rather live in their own homes than in a nursing facility or even in the home of a loved one. People with mild cognitive impairment or early-stage dementia often can function adequately in their own homes alone or with a little assistance. As the condition worsens, though, your loved one's ability to carry out simple tasks like preparing a meal or taking a bath becomes impaired. Judgment, too, is affected, and your loved one may start making unsafe decisions like smoking in bed, eating only sweets instead of nutritious foods, or climbing up into an attic while he or she is alone in the house. As your loved one's vision and balance become impaired, you may also start to notice bruises and other injuries due to frequent falls.

Eventually, the day may come when your loved one is no longer safe at home alone. If and when that day arrives, you will have to make some difficult choices about alternate living arrangements.

Until that point, you can help support your loved one's continued independence by:

Providing proper medical care. If your loved one is experiencing MCI or early-stage dementia, talk to his or her doctor about medications that might delay the onset or slow the progression of symptoms. Your loved one may also be a candidate for cognitive rehabilitation, which can also significantly slow the progression of the disease.

Providing a personal medical alarm. A personal medical alarm is a device that taps into your loved one's phone system. Your loved one wears a wireless button embedded in a necklace or a bracelet. If he or she should happen to fall or have another emergency, he or she can press the button. The device automatically connects your loved one to a call center where a technician can talk with him or her through a speaker and summon help if needed.

Hiring a caregiver. It's a good idea to hire a home caregiver to spend some time with your loved one at least a few days a week. A professional caregiver can provide many services, such as helping with meal preparation, household chores and personal care. Perhaps even more important, a caregiver can provide companionship and can encourage your loved one to get out of the house to run errands, visit the doctor or senior center, or just go for a walk around the block. Your loved one will benefit from having regular social interactions, and you will benefit from knowing that your loved one's needs are being well attended to.

Checking-in Daily. Try to make sure that you or another family member or friend call your loved one at least once a day to make sure that he or she is well and has everything he or she needs. These regular check-ins will also help you monitor your loved one's mood and cognitive status so that you can quickly react and adapt to physical, mental or emotional changes.

Providing medication set-up. People with dementia frequently have problems taking their medications as prescribed. They may have several co-existing conditions that require different medicines at different times throughout the day; this can be a lot of information to incorporate. You can help by purchasing a medication box with three or four time slots for each day of the week. Then you can stop by and fill the box once a week, making it easier for your loved one to remember to take his or her medications. A hired caregiver can also help with medication reminders.

Driving

Not everyone who has been diagnosed with dementia needs to hand over his or her car keys immediately, but there are many factors inherent in progressive dementia that make driving unsafe.

One of the most significant problems is having a delayed response time. When a healthy brain senses danger, it immediately sends out signals telling the body how to react. The brain damaged by dementia takes more time to interpret and respond to danger signals. This can cause unsafe behaviors, such as speeding through yellow lights, ignoring train signals, or going through stop signs. It can also be an issue in heavy traffic where a lot of stopping and starting is required.

Another problem with driving and dementia is poor judgment. A person may, for instance, press the accelerator instead of the brakes, shift into a lane already occupied by another vehicle, or drive much too slowly or too quickly for the road conditions.

Still one more issue of concern is the risk of your loved one getting lost, even on familiar routes.

Jack told his daughter he was taking his truck to the local grocery store, located less than a mile away from his home. He had made that trip hundreds of times. This time, however, he did not return home for hours. The police eventually found him more than 20 miles away. He was out of gas, confused and terrified. Luckily he had not been hurt, but he and his daughter decided together that his driving days were over.

If you have concerns about your loved one's driving, there are several options available to you:

Talk with your loved one. Express your concerns about his or her driving. You may find that your loved one shares those concerns. If you and your loved one agree that driving is no longer a safe option, get rid of his or her vehicle as soon as possible and arrange for other means of transportation. For instance, you could pay for a taxi to take your loved one shopping twice a week, or you could hire a caregiver who can help him or her run errands, go to doctors' appointments, attend his or her place of worship, visit the local senior center and more.

Involve your loved one's doctor. Even if your loved one is far too impaired to drive, he or she may not want to admit it. Try bringing your loved one's doctor into the conversation. Ask the doctor to write a prescription telling your loved one not to drive. The doctor can also write a letter to the Department of Motor Vehicles, asking them to require your loved one to take a driving test. If the order not to drive comes from an authority figure instead of a family member, your loved one might be more likely to follow it.

Hide or disable the car. If your loved one with dementia continues to insist upon driving, disable the car so that it won't start or move it around the block where your loved one can't see it. (For a dementia patient, out of sight is often out of mind.) If your loved one does ask about the car, say something like, "It broke down," or "It's in the shop." Then change the subject. The risk here is that your loved one may believe the car has been stolen.

Managing Finances

Managing finances can be difficult enough if you're cognitively intact. If your memory, judgment, and ability to work complex problems are impaired, such a task becomes almost impossible.

The first clue that your loved one is no longer able to handle personal finances is bills that are getting paid late or not at all. For instance, your loved one may have his or her electricity, gas, telephone, or cable turned off due to nonpayment.

Another signal that your loved one is not making wise financial decisions is purchasing a lot of merchandise from television ads, catalogues, or telemarketers. Telemarketers, especially, are usually willing to spend some time chatting with your loved one in exchange for a large sale.

Finally, be on guard if your loved one starts to make donations he or she can't afford to unfamiliar charities. Again, there's a good chance that your loved one is lonely and is being exploited by a telephone solicitor who offers conversation in exchange for donations.

If you suspect that your loved one with dementia is no longer able to handle finances, there are certain measures you can take:

Speak to your loved one. Express concern that managing the household budget has become "too stressful." Offer to help to take the responsibility off his or her shoulders or at least reduce some of the stress. If the offer is phrased in a way that doesn't shame your loved one, he or she may be grateful for the help.

Reach out to your loved one's bank. It's especially important to let your loved one's bank know if you believe your loved one is being scammed or defrauded. With your loved one's consent, you may also be able to arrange for his or her monthly bills to be paid directly from an account, removing the need for writing checks.

Contact your loved one's utility companies. Explain that your loved one has been diagnosed with dementia and sometimes forgets to pay his or her bills. Ask the companies to notify you before shutting off your loved one's service for nonpayment. This gives you time to pay the bill yourself or to remind your loved one to make a payment.

Respecting your loved one's independence while acknowledging the toll progressive dementia takes on his or her ability to function is a tough balancing act. You'll find it easier to approach your loved one as if you are trying to solve a mutual problem ("What can *we* do to make sure your power stays on this winter?"). Blaming ("How could *you* forget to pay the electric bill?") rarely gets you anywhere.

It may also help to enlist family and friends so that you are not the only one expressing concern about your loved one's ability to live alone, drive, or manage money.

Finally, consider hiring a caregiver who can observe your loved one's abilities and let you know about any changes or declines. *Tony only had time to visit his mother in the mornings when she was alert, oriented and in a good mood. The caregiver he had hired to help her during the evening hours, however, described a very different woman, a woman who was deeply confused and who often tried to get out of the house because she was looking for her mother.*

Based on that information, Tony quietly took over his mother's bookkeeping, talked her into giving the car to her oldest grandson and arranged for a full-time caregiver. His mother was able to remain safely in her home for the last nine months of her life.

Whether your loved one lives in your home or his or her own home, safety is a priority. The next chapter will discuss the potential home safety hazards that often pose a problem for people with dementia and how to manage them to make the environment as safe as possible.

CHAPTER NINE:
HAZARDS AT HOME

Most of us think of home as a safe haven—the place we feel most comfortable and at ease. For the person with dementia, though, the home can pose several hidden hazards. You can help your loved one avoid most of them by being vigilant and assessing home safety when you visit. We know, however, that it is not always possible to monitor activity 24/7—not even a nursing facility can offer that kind of supervision. No matter how closely you watch your loved one, an accident may occur. This chapter is designed to not only address potential home hazards but to also explain best practices should an injury occur.

Falls

People with dementia are often at high risk for falls. One of the most common culprits is the loss of depth perception, a problem especially seen in people with Alzheimer's disease. Poor depth perception may cause your loved one to miss the edge of a chair or a couch when sitting down or miss a step on the stairs. Similarly, difficulty in recognizing contrast can hinder the ability to see rugs with zig-zagging patterns and result in tripping and falling. You can help with this problem by providing close supervision and verbal cues such as, "Keep backing up a few more steps until you feel the chair against the backs of your legs." Depending on how advanced your loved one's dementia has become, you may need to physically help guide him or her into a safe position before giving the cue to sit down.

Another common cause of falls is dizziness or unsteadiness due to medications or weakness due to other medical conditions. If your loved one is taking atypical antipsychotics or benzodiazepines, or if he or she is experiencing weakness due to an illness like COPD, CHF or cancer, it is important that he or she stand up slowly and take a minute to steady and orient himself or herself before trying to walk. If your loved one gets too tired to remain standing while showering, you can purchase a tub bench from almost any pharmacy. This will allow your loved one to sit down during showers.

Cognitive impairments are a third reason for falls. As dementia progresses, many people forget that they need to use a cane or a walker for balance, or that they require the assistance of another person to walk. People with dementia may also get up and wander around the home at night without a flashlight—if motion-detected lights are not present in the home, your loved one can stumble in the dark, not even realizing a light switch may be nearby. If you do not sleep in the same room as your loved one, purchasing a baby monitor that will alert you to any nighttime wandering is a good investment. If you hear your loved one moving around, you can get up and either keep an eye on him or her or guide him or her safely back to bed.

Changes in balance, mobility and coordination increase chances of slipping while walking. These falls frequently occur in the kitchen or the bathroom where tile is often present and spills are common. You can reduce the likelihood of these falls by cleaning up any spills as soon as they happen and purchasing non-skid bath mats and rugs, as well as shoes or slippers with non-slip soles. Avoid letting your loved one walk around barefoot or in socks.

A pathological fracture, which occurs when your loved one's bones are fragile, can also increase fall risk. When your loved one stands up and places all weight on his or her legs, a bone in the leg can fracture under the pressure and cause a fall. Aside from making sure your loved one gets enough calcium in his or her diet, there is no way to prevent a pathological fracture from occurring.

When you are considering whether to keep your loved one at home or place him or her in a nursing or an assisted living facility, remember this: If your loved one has fallen at home, he or she is also likely to fall in a facility. A fall takes only a split second to occur, and facility staff can't monitor your loved one 24/7. If falls are your chief worry, you may be better off hiring a home caregiver who can dedicate full, 100% attention to your loved one.

If a fall does occur, there are several steps you can take to reduce the chance of serious injury, including the following:

Tell your loved one not to move. If your loved one has a broken bone, internal damage, or a head wound, moving around or struggling to get up might make things worse.

Look for noticeable bruises or breaks. Look for limbs bent at a strange angle and any areas that are bleeding. If your loved one has a significant amount of blood from a head wound, call 911 immediately. Doctors might want to perform a painless test called a CT scan to make sure that there is no internal bleeding or swelling in the brain.

Ask your loved one about pain. After a fall, it's normal for your loved one to complain of scrapes and bruises on the hands, elbows and knees. If, however, he or she reports having sharp pain in the hip or thigh, or if he or she complains of pain in the stomach or chest, it's best to call 911 and have a doctor examine your loved one. Again, the doctor might want your loved one to undergo a CT scan of the chest and abdomen to make sure there is no internal bleeding.

Check for range of motion (ROM). This involves taking each arm and leg and gently bending and extending it. Move slowly and stop at once if your loved one cries out or complains of sharp or piercing pain.

Help your loved one sit up. Once you have checked your loved one over and are reasonably sure that there are no serious injuries, help him sit or her up in a comfortable position.

Use a gait belt to help your loved one stand. A gait belt is a belt that fastens around your loved one's waist. Using a gait belt to help your loved one stand is much safer for both of you than pulling on his or her arms. Crouch down to your loved one's level and instruct him or her to bend the knees so that his or her feet are resting flat against the floor. Instruct your loved one to push against the ground with his or her feet. At the same time, pull up on the gait belt. Be sure to use your legs to lift and not your back.

Call for help if you can't get your loved one up safely. If your loved one is unable to push with his or her legs, you may need to call another household member or a neighbor to help you get your loved one off the floor. Another option is to call 911. The paramedics will help your loved one off the floor and check him or her over. While you wait for help to arrive, do what you can to make your loved one comfortable. For instance, you might want to cover your loved one with a blanket or put a pillow under his or her head. Don't scold your loved one for falling, even if the fall was his "fault."

Burns and Scalds

Burns occur when your loved one's skin comes into contact with a hot object, such as a burner on the stove. Scalds occur when your loved one's skin comes into contact with a hot fluid, such as boiling liquids or bathwater that is running at too high a temperature.

Most burns and scalds occur in the kitchen or the bathroom. You can help prevent them by supervising your loved one. If your loved one wants to help you cook, ask him or her to assist with tasks that do not involve being near the oven. Safe tasks include making a salad, setting the table, polishing silverware (not the knives), shelling walnuts, and decorating cookies or cupcakes.

When your loved one is in the kitchen, turn the handles of all the pots and pans so that they are facing the wall instead of facing outward. This makes it less likely that your loved one will grab the handle of a hot pan and tip the contents over on himself or herself.

Finally, ask your plumber to lower the thermostat on your water so that the temperature doesn't become too hot. Since dementia slows reaction time, some people scald themselves by stepping into a bath that is too hot and not getting out quickly enough to prevent serious damage.

If your loved one receives a burn or a scald wound, there are several treatments you can apply:

Remove from the source of the burn. Quickly pull your loved one's body part away from the hot surface or dry off the hot liquid.

Do not remove any clothing stuck to the burn. It's a good idea to remove jewelry and clothing that are around the area of the burn, but do not remove any clothing that has adhered to the burned skin. Doing so could cause more damage.

Apply cool (not cold) or lukewarm water to the burned area. Cool or lukewarm water will ease the pain and minimize the damage caused by the burn. If possible, use water running from a tap. If not, get a large pot or bucket, fill it with cool water, and immerse the burned spot.

Do not apply greasy substances like butter. The idea that putting butter or another greasy substance like Crisco on a burn will help the burn heal faster is an old wives' tale. In fact, these substances may make the burn worse.

Keep your loved one calm. Wrap a blanket around your loved one's shoulders to keep him or her warm and to help prevent shock. It also helps if you talk to your loved one in a gentle, reassuring voice. Make conversation and encourage your loved one to answer your questions.

Apply a clean gauze dressing. Apply a loose gauze dressing, making sure to tape around the burn and not directly on it.

There are some situations when it's best to take your loved one directly to the hospital for medical attention. In fact, you should always take someone over the age of 60 to the emergency room unless the burn is extremely minor. Some other cases where immediate medical attention is recommended include:

- Large burns—bigger than the size of your loved one's hand
- Deep burns—skin appears white or charred
- Blistered burns that occur on the face, hands, arms, feet, legs, or genitals
- When other health conditions like lung disease, heart disease or cancer are present

Elopement

Most people associate the word elopement with a "secret marriage," but by definition elopement also simply means to run away. In the context of dementia, elopement refers to the situation where your loved one may wander away from the home without your knowledge. Elopement can be intentional or accidental.

In the intentional case, your loved one may leave to search for something or someone, such as a parent or a childhood home. Before this kind of elopement occurs, your loved one may seem anxious or ask repetitive questions ("Where is my mother? Have you seen my mother?"). Your loved one may also complain of you keeping him in the house against his or her will ("What's the matter with you? I have to go to work."). If you notice these potential warning signs, try to reassure your loved one that all is well and that he or she is in exactly the right place.

Elopement may also be unintentional. Sometimes, the person with dementia forgets the layout of the home, even if he or she has occupied that home for years. While wandering aimlessly around the house, the person may find a door to the outside and walk through it. Once outside, he or she can become lost, confused, and unable to find the way back in.

A similar accidental case of elopement occurs when a person with dementia goes outside for a specific purpose, such as to take out the trash and then cannot remember which house is his or hers.

Amanda loved to look at the newspaper in the mornings and waited eagerly for the paper boy to toss it on the sidewalk. One morning, she went out to get the paper and couldn't remember which house was hers. The weather was quite cold, and Amanda was wearing only a nightgown, a robe and some slippers. Luckily, a neighbor spotted her halfway down the block and ran out to intercept her. Amanda explained that she didn't know where she was supposed to go. "All the houses look alike," she wept.

Elopement can be difficult to prevent, especially if your loved one is determined to find a way outside. There are, however, some things you can do to make it less likely:

Buy a baby monitor. This allows you to listen to your loved one's activities at night. If he or she gets out of bed and starts moving around, you can provide supervision and redirection until your loved one is ready to go back to sleep.

Place alarms on your outside doors. Electronic stores often carry simple door alarms that sound an alert every time the door is opened. The alarm serves two purposes: the sudden noise startles the person with dementia and makes him or her less likely to approach the door again; the sound also alerts you that your loved one is near a door leading outside so that you can intervene to keep him or her safe.

Put extra locks on outside doors. Place an extra latch-hook or a chain-link lock significantly above or below your loved one's line of vision. When the door doesn't open easily, your loved one will usually give up and walk away.

Disguise doors to the outside. Buy a roll of wallpaper that looks like a bookshelf or the inside of a kitchen cabinet. Your loved one may not even realize a door is there.

Post a warning sign on the door. You can use your computer to create a large red stop sign, or a sign that reads, "Danger! Do NOT Enter!" You may have to be creative based on your loved one's background. One particular gentleman, for instance, had spent his entire life employed by a large corporation. His loved ones found that he stayed away from outside doors when they posted signs that read, "SHHH...Meeting in progress. Do not disturb." Another woman who had taken many trips with her husband stayed away from doors that read, "Pilots only beyond this point."

If wandering occurs, there are measures you can take to help bring your loved one home quickly. The first is to enroll your loved one in the Medic Alert® + Alzheimer's Safe Return® program in the United States. This is a nationwide program that provides bracelets for people who may wander. The bracelet is engraved with a unique identification number and a toll-free number to a call center. If a law enforcement official or anyone else finds your loved one wandering, they will contact the call center, and the call center will contact you. For more information, contact the local chapter of your Alzheimer's Association or visit **http://www.alz.org**.

Canada has a similar program called the Safely Home Registry. The program varies from province to province. You can find out more by getting in touch with your local chapter of the Alzheimer Society or by visiting Safely Home at **http://www.safelyhome.ca/**.

Call the police as soon as you realize your loved one is missing. Explain to them that your loved one has a diagnosis of dementia and may be lost and unable to remember even the most basic information such as his or her name. It's also a good idea to keep a current picture of your loved one on hand at all times.

You can help by canvasing the neighborhood and speaking to neighbors who might have seen your loved one. It's a good idea to check with local hospitals to see if they are treating any "unknown" elderly patients.

If your loved one goes missing and the police become involved, the situation will probably be reported to the agency handling adult protective services (APS) in your state. This is a routine referral. Try to avoid becoming upset or defensive. APS workers know that it can be very difficult to stop people with dementia from eloping. Unless the situation at the home where your loved one lives is clearly abusive or neglectful, they will not try to remove your loved one from your care. Quite the opposite, they may be able to offer some pointers and resources that can help you keep your loved one safe.

Scams

Just because you wouldn't take advantage of an elderly, confused person doesn't mean that there aren't plenty of people who are more than willing to do just that.

Con artists usually make contact by phone, although if your loved one gets online, there are plenty of scammers on the Internet as well. Con artists usually avoid using direct mail for scams because using the mail service with the intent to defraud carries federal penalties.

Con artists know that many elderly people worry about their finances and leaving money for their children and grandchildren. Thus, the most typical scams perpetrated on the elderly include

- Worthless investments
- Collecting taxes for a "grand prize" your loved one has presumably won
- Offering "collectibles" guaranteed to gain in value

Most con artists start out by pretending to be friendly and sympathetic. They make common cause with your loved one ("You remind me so much of one of my family members"), and they'll listen to your loved one tell stories, even if repetitive.

Then, slowly, the pressure begins to build. "I like you, and I'd like to make you a very rich person, but first I need your credit card number." If gentle persuasion doesn't work, the pressure may escalate. "I guess you're too senile to understand that I'm giving you a once in a lifetime opportunity," or "Your son will probably put you in a nursing home when he hears about the chance you just passed up."

Already confused, and now upset by the cruel words of his or her new friend, your loved one may very well give in and provide account information just to stop the attack. Sadly, once your loved one has fallen for one scam, the name and phone number will be placed on a list targeting him or her for other scams.

Dementia may keep some people from realizing that they are actually being taken advantage of. Even if your loved one does suspect this is the case, he or she may not tell you about these troubles for fear that you really will consider placement in a nursing home. Even if your loved one cannot fully explain what is happening due to language difficulties, there may be other signs that suggest he or she is being scammed.

- The phone rings frequently when you visit, but the caller hangs up if you answer.
- Your loved one's bank or checking account shows large charges to companies you don't recognize.
- You notice many new, low-quality gadgets in your loved one's home. (These are often the "grand prizes.")

If you see any of these warning signs, try the following interventions.

Approach your loved one kindly and sensitively. Rather than making angry accusations, you might say, "Mom, I've been hearing from friends that a lot of their parents are getting calls from people who are trying to take advantage of them. Has this happened to you?"

If you can confirm that a scam or a fraud has occurred, report it to the authorities.

Place your loved one's phone number on the "Do Not Call Registry." In the United States, call **1-888-382-1222** from your loved one's phone. In Canada, this is known as the "National Do Not Call List." The phone number to register is **1-866-580-3625**.

Hire a home caregiver. This will help in two ways. First, it will mean that someone is in your loved one's home on a regular basis to monitor for suspicious calls. Second, a caregiver will provide your loved one with the needed socialization and friendship so he or she does not have to make friends with con artists.

Assist with your loved one's finances. Offer to take over paying the bills and balancing the bank book so your loved one doesn't have to worry about this burden. If your loved one still wants to be involved in financial decisions, suggest that you get together once or twice a month to go over bills and statements together. You and your loved one may also want to consider canceling credit cards so they cannot be misused.

Abuse and Neglect

Physical abuse involves doing something to deliberately cause your loved one bodily pain or injury. This might include slapping, burning, punching, kicking, or deliberately grabbing your loved one's arm tightly enough to cause bruises.

Emotional abuse involves a pattern of saying hurtful, demeaning things that threaten your loved one's mental wellbeing. It can include shouting, threats, name-calling, and insults. We all lose our tempers once in a while and say things we wish we hadn't, but the emotionally abusive caregiver repeatedly uses words to purposefully damage self-esteem.

Financial abuse involves deliberately misusing the assets of the person with dementia to the caregiver's own benefit.

When Alan felt "stuck" with the care of his mother, for instance, he placed her in a senior high rise, took all but a few dollars of her social security check each month, and disappeared until the first of the next month when he would arrive to collect the social security money once again. His behavior came to light when his mother started knocking on her neighbors' doors asking for food. The courts removed Alan's power in any and all decisions involving his mother and appointed a guardian to make sure his mother was receiving proper care as well as a conservator to look after his mother's money.

Sexual abuse involves rape, touching the victim's genitals, or forcing the victim to touch the perpetrator's genitals. It can also involve sexual remarks and unwanted propositions.

Neglect involves not providing adequate food, shelter, clothing, and care. In the scenario above, Alan was neglectful as well as financially abusive because he did not leave his mother enough money to buy food.

Sadly, people with Alzheimer's disease and related dementias often become victims of abuse and neglect. This can happen for several reasons. People with dementia often exhibit troubling or offensive behaviors. They may say rude things to their caregivers or create messes around the house. It is the caregiver's point of view that ultimately determines whether abuse or neglect occurs. If the caregiver realizes that his or her loved one is not at fault and would not say such horrible things if it weren't for the dementia, then the caregiver probably will not become abusive. If the caregiver believes, however, that the loved one is choosing to behave badly, abuse and neglect are more likely to occur.

As Anna's dementia progressed, she started to become incontinent. Embarrassed by her wet, dirty clothes, she often hid them around the house instead of putting them in the laundry hamper. Anna's caregiver, her daughter, believed that Anna was just hiding the clothes to make extra work for her. She started shouting at her mother and sometimes even shaking her. A neighbor saw this and reported the matter to APS. Anna's daughter was placed in a class for dementia caregivers where she learned that her mother's behavior was not unusual and was caused by the disease, not intention.

Another factor in abuse or neglect is the caregiver's past relationship with his or her loved one. Some children who were abused, for instance, may end up as caregivers and abuse the elder as a form of payback.

Like many other types of abuse, the abuse of people with dementia tends to escalate over time. Intervention is most likely to help in the earliest stages of abuse or neglect.

If you feel as if you are getting close to abusing or neglecting your loved one, get help right away. Call APS, or reach out to the Alzheimer's Association or the Alzheimer Society. If stress is a factor, try hiring a part-time caregiver who can keep your loved one company while you get out of the house, take a bath, or shut yourself in the bedroom with a good book—respite is important for your mental and physical wellbeing.

If you are not the primary caregiver but you witness the primary caregiver being abusive towards your loved one, confront him or her tactfully but directly. ("Please don't yell at Dad like that. He doesn't understand what he is doing.") Brainstorm with the primary caregiver to remove some of the stress. Perhaps you could offer to provide care one day a week. If you don't have the time to provide care yourself, offer to contribute towards hiring a professional caregiver who can give the primary caregiver a break. Finally, keep a close eye on the situation. If you suspect abuse or neglect has continued, call APS.

One of the most effective ways of managing your loved one's problem behaviors is learning to communicate efficiently with him or her. The next chapter looks at communication issues and best practices to overcome them.

CHAPTER TEN:
COMMUNICATION

How you go about communicating with your loved one can make a big difference in how he or she thinks, feels, and behaves. There are several theories about the ideal way to interact with people with dementia, and all have their pros and cons. You may choose to use just one technique or a combination of several. It all depends on your preferences, your loved one's personality and the stage of the dementia.

Whatever approach you select, it's important to make sure that your loved one is listening to you. When you have something important to say, turn off other sources of sound, such as the television or radio. Stand directly in front of your loved one, or crouch beside his or her chair, and make direct eye contact. Then speak slowly using simple words and sentences.

If the message you are delivering is a complex one or one that is likely to cause an emotional reaction, speak one sentence at a time and make sure your loved one understands what you have said before you continue.

Reality Orientation

Reality orientation involves reminding your loved one of his or her name and identity, the date and time, and the place.

Thomas has a chalkboard in his room that reads, *"My name is Thomas Jones. I am a mechanic. I worked for TWA for 20 years. I live with my son, Mitch, in Topeka Kansas."*

There are several tools that can help orient your loved one to reality. These include a chalkboard, like Thomas has in his room, a large clock, a large calendar, or a map.

Studies suggest that reality orientation is correlated with improvements in cognition and behavior. It seems to be most effective with people whose dementia is in the early stages. It also works best when it is used in a passive manner, such as placing a large calendar with the date circled on your loved one's door, instead of a confrontational such as telling a loved one who is looking for his mother, "Look at the date, Dad. You're 85 years old, and your mother has been dead for years." Confrontations not only result in feelings of confusion but also sadness.

It often works best to orient your loved one in the morning before the confusion of the day begins. For instance, when Mitch knocks on Thomas's door in the morning, he always says something like, "Good morning, Dad. It's me, Mitch, your son. Today is Tuesday and it's 8:00 a.m. and time for breakfast."

Validation Therapy

Validation therapy, pioneered by Naomi Feil, MSW, ACSW, emphasizes acceptance of the emotional reality and personal truth of another person. Rather than arguing about facts, the validation therapy model recommends acknowledging and engaging with your loved one's thoughts and feelings.

For instance, if your father states in March, "It will be Christmas soon," a validating response might be, "What got you thinking about Christmas?" or "What is your favorite thing about Christmas?"

The chief benefit of validation therapy is improving communication skills. This benefit can be attributed to the non-confrontational nature of validation therapy. The person with dementia is not constantly being told that he or she is "wrong" and is not continually subjected to information that challenges his or her own notions of reality. Such support encourages the exchange of thoughts, concerns and desires. It is common, however, for family members to feel uncomfortable with this approach, as it can feel like a deliberate deception. Remind yourself that your actions are for the betterment of your loved one's psychological and emotional well-being.

Therapeutic Deception

Therapeutic deception refers to the practice of telling a "little white lie" that might be less painful for your loved one to hear than the truth.

Comfort level with this technique varies from one person to another. If you can wrap your head around the idea that honesty may not always be the best policy, you may occasionally find deception a useful communication tool. If not, use one of the other strategies suggested in this chapter that you feel more relaxed practicing.

When Caroline's family decided it was time to place her in a nursing home, they did not tell her that the new living arrangement would be permanent. They felt she was too confused to understand the information and would probably soon forget it, anyway. Instead, they told her the doctor wanted her to stay in the facility "for a little while." During the first week or two, Caroline asked repeatedly when she would be allowed to go home. Within a month, however, she had forgotten she'd ever lived anywhere else. In this case, therapeutic deception spared her the pain of grieving for her lost home.

Instructions and Verbal Cues

As dementia progresses, a large portion of your communications with your loved one will involve providing instructions and verbal cues about how to perform a specific task. Sometimes, it may seem easier to just complete the task for your loved one yourself —for instance, to dress your loved one rather than to wait while he or she dresses himself or herself. It's important, however, to encourage your loved one to complete tasks that he or she is still capable of doing to support independence and physical and psychological health but also to slow cognitive decline.

When giving instructions, it is important to keep a few tips in mind:

1. **Use short sentences.** Instead of saying, "First I want you to pick up the shirt on your bed," simply say, "Pick up the shirt."

2. **Take it one step at a time.** Don't string a list of orders together– "Now button your shirt, put on your socks, put on your shoes, and tie the laces." Start with one task at a time.

3. **Give your loved one time to follow your instructions.** Dementia slows the speed with which the brain processes speech. It also slows reaction time. Thus, it is important that you allow time for your loved one to understand your request before moving on to the next step. If a few minutes have gone by and your loved one seems stuck, repeat the instruction clearly and gently touch the part of his body that needs to be moved. For instance, lightly tap your loved one's right hand and say, "Pick up your shirt."

4. **Allow plenty of time.** A sense of urgency will make your loved one even more confused and stressed. If you have an appointment, help your loved one get ready early.

Redirection

Redirection (see Chapter 13) can be a useful tool if your loved one becomes fixated on a certain thought or behavior or becomes particularly irritated and frustrated. At its most basic level, redirection simply means changing the subject or introducing a new activity—in a sense, distracting the person from the situation or thought that may be troubling him or her. Ideally, redirection will touch on your loved one's deepest interests.

Elizabeth had loved cats her entire life. Though she no longer recognized her family members, she could recall every cat she'd ever had. Sometimes in the afternoon, she became anxious and called out, "Help me, help me." Her granddaughter could always calm her by snuggling up beside her on the couch and saying, "Tell me about your first cat, Grandma Liz." As Elizabeth got involved in the story, she quickly forgot her anxiety.

Nonverbal Communication

In face-to-face conversations between two cognitively intact people, some researchers suggest body language makes up approximately 55% of what we communicate to each other. The tone and pitch of our voices comprises around 38% of our communication. The actual words we choose only contribute about 7% of what we communicate.

Nonverbal communication is especially important in dementia care because your loved one will likely lose her ability to speak and understand language at some point. Nonverbal cues may become the ideal and only way you can assess your loved one's needs and wants and express your own thoughts and feelings.

People in late-stage dementia, especially those with Parkinson's-type dementia, often lose the ability to control their facial muscles resulting in a persistent mask-like facial expression, devoid of smiling or frowning. Furthermore, the body often becomes tense or rigid due to the disease process. These changes can impede your ability to read emotions from your loved one's facial movements and body signals. You can still, however, identify anxiety or unhappiness by observing your loved one's movements for cues like wringing his or her hands, repeatedly tapping a foot, pulling away from touch, or wrapping his or her arms around himself or herself as a form of self-comfort.

You can also use nonverbal communication to relate to your loved one—a smile, a comforting arm around the shoulders, a manicure, a handclasp, or cuddling under a warm blanket may all be welcome signs of affection. Again, you can rely on your loved one's body language to let you know which kinds of touch are welcome and which are not.

A large part of dementia care is learning the many different ways to communicate effectively with your loved one. The next chapter will discuss how you can assist your loved one with activities of daily living such as getting dressed, feeding, bathing, and going to the bathroom.

CHAPTER ELEVEN:
DEMENTIA AND PERSONAL CARE

The tasks that make up daily self-care, such as taking a bath or shower, getting dressed, eating a meal, and taking ourselves to the bathroom are called activities of daily living (ADLs).

The tasks that allow us to live independently but are not necessary for basic functioning such as balancing a budget, shopping at the grocery store, and completing housework are called instrumental activities of daily living (IADLs).

As dementia worsens, it compromises your loved one's ability to perform both ADLs and IADLs. IADLs become difficult first, although interventions like cognitive rehabilitation, performed as a part of Dementia Therapeutics™, can help people maintain and even relearn these skills.

As your loved one's dementia progresses to middle- and late-stage, his or her ability to care for himself or herself through basic ADLs becomes impaired. At this point, your loved one is usually unable to live alone without some sort of assistance and supervision. This chapter discusses several ways in which you can help your loved one with personal care.

Maintain Independence as Long as Possible

Most people are able to manage some ADLs until quite late in the dementia process, as long as they have someone standing by to offer verbal instructions and supervision (See Chapter Ten for tips on offering instructions effectively). Again, it's important to encourage your loved one to complete the ADLs he or she is still able to do independently or with limited assistance, even if it takes more time and patience on your part.

First, being able to complete self-care rituals like washing one's hands or buttoning one's shirt gives your loved one a sense of accomplishment, promoting what mental health professionals call self-efficacy. It feels much better to be able to take care of yourself than to have to rely on someone else for the most basic kinds of care.

Second, the more you challenge your loved one to use the cognitive skills he or she has remaining, the longer those skills will last—when dealing with the brain, "Use it or lose it," is a true statement.

Finally, the more your loved one can do for himself or herself, the greater the likelihood that you will be able to keep him or her in a home setting longer.

Unfortunately, Alzheimer's disease and many other forms of dementia are progressive. The time will come when your loved one will have to depend on a caregiver for physical assistance in completing all of his or her ADLs. If you are that caregiver, there are several things you can do to put your loved one at ease:

Maintain Privacy and Dignity

No matter how cognitively impaired your loved one may be, he or she is still capable of feeling humiliated if personal care is not handled sensitively. You should treat your loved one with the respect an adult deserves.

Make sure to keep your loved one's private parts covered in front of other family members or friends. If you are taking your loved one into the bathroom for a bath or a shower, make sure she is wrapped in a thick robe or wait until you get him or her into the bathroom to begin removing his or her clothes.

If you are giving a bed bath, use towels and bed clothes to cover, or drape, the parts of the body that are not being washed. This not only minimizes exposure, it can also help keep your loved one warm and comfortable.

Adopt a calm, matter-of-fact manner during personal care. If you convey with your body language, tone of voice, and words that there is no reason to be embarrassed, your loved one is more likely to be relaxed and less likely to resist care.

Finally, don't make any mention of the personal care once you have completed it. Be especially careful to avoid shaming statements like, "You should be grateful to me! I wipe your bottom, you know."

If you are not comfortable providing personal care to your loved one, or if you sense your loved one is uncomfortable receiving care from you (this dynamic may be especially evident between a mother and an adult son), consider hiring a professional caregiver. Sometimes, it is easier to accept care from a neutral, skilled caregiver than from a family member.

Incontinence

Lena lived at home with her daughter, Ann. As her dementia progressed, Lena began losing control of her bladder and bowels. Embarrassed, she removed her soiled clothes and hid them under her bed or at the back of her closet. When Ann confronted Lena with the garments, Lena angrily denied that the clothes were hers. (By that time, she probably didn't remember that they were.)

Like Lena, people with dementia often develop incontinence as their disease gets worse. Women tend to try to hide the problem while men may be more open and start urinating in inappropriate places like trash cans or house plants.

There are no perfect ways to address the problem of incontinence, but there are some strategies that might help, such as:

Clothes that fasten in back. This kind of clothing, developed especially for people with dementia, can prevent problems like undressing in public or urinating in public places. The problem with this kind of clothing is that people wearing it cannot go to the bathroom without the assistance of a caregiver. People with dementia may also find clothes that fasten in back confusing and frustrating.

Adult briefs. Adult briefs are disposable padded underwear that people put on just as they would put on ordinary panties or boxers. The padding protects the outer clothing in the event of an accident, and if the briefs become wet or soiled, they can be thrown away. The main problem with adult briefs is that some people with dementia don't like wearing them. They may feel bulky and uncomfortable, and some people are offended by the idea of wearing a "diaper."

Adult diapers. Disposable adult diapers, most commonly used for people who are confined to bed or a wheelchair, are placed and fastened just like a diaper worn by an infant. Like adult briefs, they provide effective protection for outer clothing and most people who require them are too cognitively impaired to object.

Disposable bed pads. Known informally as "chux," these pads are placed underneath your loved one on top of the fitted sheet or mattress (if fitted sheet is not being used). They are usually used in conjunction with adult briefs or adult diapers to keep your loved one's mattress clean and dry. They are especially useful for people who are bedbound.

Perineal care. The perineum is the area on your loved one's body located between the genitals and the anus. If it is not kept clean and dry, it can become irritated and develop a painful rash. When your loved one is incontinent, it is important to use—or coach your loved one to use—a moistened cloth to clean urine and feces away from the perineal area. Your loved one's doctor may also suggest using powder or cream to further protect your loved one's skin.

The Principles of Standby Assistance

There are several different levels of care that you may be called upon to provide to your loved one. Standby assistance requires proper preparation, verbal cues, and lending a helping hand when necessary.

For instance, if you were helping your father transfer from his wheelchair to bed, standby assistance might look something like this:

1. Position the wheelchair at a 90-degree angle to the bed.
2. Lock the wheelchair's brakes.
3. Release the footrests and swing them out of the way so your father won't trip over them.
4. Make sure your father is wearing shoes or slippers with non-slip soles.

5. Ask your father to plant his feet flat on the ground and his hands on the armrests of the wheelchair.
6. Ask him to stand by pushing up with his hands and feet.
7. Use a gait belt for leverage and assistance as needed.
8. Tell your father to pivot until he feels the mattress against the backs of his legs.
9. Use the gait belt as needed to maneuver him into the correct position.
10. Instruct him to sit down on the mattress.
11. Instruct him to swing his legs onto the bed, providing assistance as needed.

As you can see, most of the physical help you offer during this process is minor and focuses more on supporting and steadying your loved one than on using your own strength to help with things like lifting and turning.

A smaller caregiver is usually capable of offering standby assistance to a larger loved one.

The Principles of Total Assistance

If your loved one is physically or cognitively unable to handle simple tasks like standing or pivoting on his or her own, she is said to need total assistance. If you are larger than your loved one, you may be able to handle the care manually with a gait belt and the use of proper body mechanics—though you would still be at increased risk for back strains and other types of injury. If you are smaller than your loved one, or if you can't maneuver him or her physically, you may need to enlist a second caregiver or use a mechanical device like a Hoyer lift. A Hoyer lift is used to transfer people who cannot bear weight. It features two legs on wheels, a large hook, and a pneumatic lifting device. A sling is placed underneath your loved one and fastened to the hook. The device is then able to lift the person and transfer him or her to a bed, wheelchair, or commode.

If your loved one is bedbound, you will need to change his or her position in bed to avoid bedsores. You can do this by using a draw sheet. This is a sheet positioned under your loved one's hips, back, and shoulders. You can use it to roll your loved one from side to side in bed. (You will probably need to tuck pillows behind his or her back and knees to help him or her hold the position.) You can also use it to move your loved one's head nearer to the top of the bed if he or she slips down.

Taking care of a loved one who requires total care can be emotionally as well as physically draining. It's a good idea to enlist a friend or family member or to hire a professional caregiver to give you a break for at least a day or two each week. You won't be able to provide optimal care to your loved one if you are not at your best. Taking time to ensure your own physical and mental health will benefit both you and your loved one.

CHAPTER TWELVE:
BEHAVIOR ISSUES

It's not uncommon for people with dementia to exhibit various behavior problems, including resistance to care, inappropriate conduct in public, or aggression. Remember, though, that many behavioral issues are the result of confusion and miscommunication—your loved one has not developed these challenging behaviors just to upset you.

This chapter looks at some of the most common behavior issues among people with dementia. It examines why they may occur and some techniques you can use to either reduce or stop them.

If you find yourself completely out of patience, don't take it out on your loved one. Go into another room for a few minutes —assuming it is safe to leave your loved one alone—and return when you feel more in control. By that time, your loved one may have stopped the troubling behavior on his or her own.

Resistance to Care

Resistance to care is any kind of behavior that makes providing personal care difficult. Some people may shout at their caregivers while others slap at their hands or try to pinch. This behavior typically appears in middle-stage dementia and fades away as the disease progresses.

People with dementia may become resistant to care if they are embarrassed, for instance if a male caregiver tries to help a female bathe or change clothes. The person with dementia may also become upset if the care is not adequately explained to him or her.

The following actions should help minimize resistance:

Tell your loved one exactly what you are going to do before you do it. Even if you do not think he or she is listening or can understand you, stand or crouch directly in front of him or her, maintain eye contact, be sure you have his or her attention, and tell him or her what to expect. Refer to body parts by their proper names.

Encourage your loved one to participate. For instance, if you are going to brush his or her teeth, say something like, "You can help me by opening your mouth as wide as you can."

Offer something to distract your loved one during care. Put on some lively music, engage your loved one in conversation if he or she is still able to talk, or give him or her some family pictures to look at.

Talk about something your loved one can look forward to when the care is complete. Examples include a dish of ice cream, a television show, or a drive around the neighborhood.

Praise your loved one. Thank your loved one for his or her cooperation (even if he or she didn't cooperate). Tell your loved one how nice he or she looks.

Repetitive Questions and Comments

Repetitive questions and comments are typical in early- to middle-stage dementia, though in some cases, the behavior might last well into the late-stage.

Your loved one doesn't mean to be annoying by incessantly repeating the same question or statement over and over. He or she is simply trying to connect with you or express a need. The damage to the part of the brain that controls short-term memory prevents your loved one from recalling that he or she said the same thing just a few seconds before and received a response. Here are some things you can do to help stop the broken-record effect:

Listen and respond to the remark. For instance, each time your father asks, "What time is it?" politely tell him the time. This approach is always appropriate, but it requires the patience of a saint—a trait most of us lack.

Use memory cues. Your father who always wants to know the time, for instance, may be satisfied by a large clock. If your loved one expresses anxiety about missing work, post a large sign in his or her room that says, "No work today!"

Look for the feelings behind the statements. For instance, if your loved one is constantly asking about the condition of his or her farm, you might respond, "You really miss living on that farm, don't you? Why don't you tell me what it was like growing up there?"

Redirect. Pick a topic or activity that you know will interest your loved one and draw attention there (for activity ideas, see Chapter 13).

Sexual Acting Out

Sexual acting out can include making inappropriate remarks about another person, touching or groping, or exposing oneself or self-stimulating in public. Only a small percentage of people with dementia have a problem with sexual acting out, but when it occurs, it can be very distressing to their loved ones.

Such behavior can occur for many reasons. First, we are all sexual beings, no matter what our age. Sexuality is a normal and healthy life function. As dementia damages the brain, however, your loved one may not know how to share sexual feelings appropriately—judgment and reasoning become impaired.

Other people who start to undress in public may not have sexual motives at all. They may be too warm or they may be looking for a place to use the bathroom. Finally, some people with dementia may confuse a stranger with a spouse or a partner.

Doris had lost her beloved husband, Michael, to a stroke three years earlier. Now living in a nursing home and suffering from middle-stage dementia, Doris met another resident named Mike. She began to get him mixed up in her head with her late husband. Neither Mike nor Doris's family was especially pleased when Doris began snuggling up to Mike in the patient lounge. Since both families objected to the relationship, the staff decided to address it using reality orientation. Whenever Doris came into the lounge and started looking for Mike, a staff member would hurry over and introduce Doris to "Mike Hadley, a librarian (Doris's husband had been a truck driver). His wife Cheryl lives across town." It took a lot of repetition, but Doris finally came to understand that Michael and Mike were two different people.

If your loved one begins acting out sexually, try these interventions:

Use reality orientation. "I'm your daughter, Holly, and you're my dad. Dads and daughters don't touch that way."

Offer plenty of caring, non-sexual touch. Your loved one may be suffering from skin hunger or lack of human contact. Making sure that he or she gets plenty of appropriate touch like non-sexual hugs and hand-holding can put a stop to the sexual acting out.

Ignore off-color comments. Change the subject—redirect.

Check for comfort. Your loved one may be undressing because he or she is too warm, his or her clothes are too tight, or he or she has to go to the bathroom.

Allow your loved one privacy to take care of sexual needs, such as masturbation.

Offer a brief, polite explanation to bystanders if behavior occurs in public. "Please excuse my mother. She has dementia."

Verbal Aggression

Verbal aggression can manifest as shouting, cursing, insulting, name-calling, and threatening others. This behavior is common in Pick's disease and other dementias that mainly affect the frontal lobe of the brain. Because that location governs impulse control, significant damage prevents your loved one from following the age-old rule, "Think before you speak." As a result, your loved one may say exactly what comes into his mind, even if it is hurtful or inappropriate.

The best response to verbal aggression is **no response**. Pretend you did not hear the offensive remark. Other tactics that help include:

Reduce the amount of stimulation. Over-stimulation can be frustrating for your loved one, and it can lead to verbal attacks. Make sure your loved one's space is calm and quiet.

Redirect your loved one. Get him or her involved in an activity like playing with a pet, stirring a cake mix, or telling a favorite story.

Encourage your loved one to take a nap. People with dementia who are over-tired often have explosive outbursts. Encourage your loved one to rest, or give him or her a few moments alone —as long as it is safe—so that he or she can calm down.

Get support for yourself. It can be frustrating to provide care for a loved one who says unkind things to you. Join a caregiver support group or hire a professional caregiver for a few days a week so that you can take a break.

Behavior problems can compound the stress you already feel in taking on the responsibilities of caregiving. It may help to remind yourself that the behavior is a symptom of the dementia, just like memory loss or disorientation. If your loved one wasn't sick, he or she wouldn't be acting that way or saying those things to you.

One way to deal with challenging behavior is to redirect your loved one and get him interested in another activity. The next chapter offers 25 all-purpose activities your loved one may enjoy.

CHAPTER THIRTEEN:
25 ACTIVITIES AND EXERCISES

Throughout this book, you've read the word "redirection" quite often, largely as a communication method of reducing agitation, confusion and fixation. Again, redirection refers to changing the subject or distracting your loved one with a new focus of attention.

Oscar, who was experiencing early-stage dementia, lived with his adult son. He appeared sad and moody. He didn't speak to anyone unless they spoke to him first, and even then his answers were as brief as possible. Although he was capable of walking, he spent all of his time lying in bed watching television. His son hired a caregiver to keep him company. After several visits, she learned that Oscar enjoyed reading. Whenever he got in one of his bad moods, she would read chapters from his favorite books aloud to him. After that, Oscar was almost always in a better mood and was willing to get up and get dressed.

One way to redirect your loved one is to introduce a new activity. This chapter offers 25 ideas you can use to keep your loved one busy, involved in family life and happy. Of course, not every suggestion is appropriate for every person, so choose ideas that fit with the personality of your loved one.

You may find that you don't have time to involve your loved one in new activities. If this is the case, you may consider hiring a private duty caregiver. New activities help the caregiver get acquainted with your loved one, and your loved one learns to associate the caregiver's visits with having a pleasant time.

These ideas will get you started, but as you read, feel free to try new activities that you think your loved one might enjoy.

1. **Walk around the block.** This is a great activity for someone who has extra nervous energy. As you walk, draw your loved one's attention to all of the interesting things you see outside —animals, trees, flowers.

2. **Build a snowman.** If the weather cooperates and your loved one is physically able, dress him or her warmly and go play in the snow. This activity may spark fun memories from your loved one's childhood that he or she can talk about later.

3. **Go fishing.** It's a quiet activity that won't over-stimulate your loved one. Catching a fish that the family can eat for dinner will also give him or her a sense of pride and accomplishment.

4. **Rake the yard in the fall.** If your loved one's coordination is questionable, you can take control and rake the leaves into piles. Ask your loved one to place them into plastic bags.

5. **Plant a garden.** Give your loved one his or her own plot of land and help him or her plant their favorite flowers. When the garden grows, you'll be able to pick fresh flowers to adorn the home and to create beautiful arrangements that can be given to friends and family.

6. **Assign your loved one an ongoing task.** Setting the table before each meal, feeding the dog, or watering the houseplants are all good ideas.

7. **Get your loved one a pet.** Being around a cat or a dog can lower your loved one's heart rate and blood pressure and release chemicals in the brain that elevate mood.

8. **Give a manicure or a pedicure.** If your loved one is female, offer her several different colors of nail polish including fun ones like hot pink and bright glittery blue.

9. **Ask your loved one to brush your hair.** It will make both of you feel good.

10. **Play simple games that can enhance memory and focus.** Ideas include Old Maid, Concentration, Uno, Battleship and Checkers. Involve as many family members in the games as possible and divide into teams. This way, if your loved one loses track of what's going on, he or she has their team to rely upon.

11. **Work a jigsaw puzzle.** Choose a picture, that once put together, your loved one will enjoy.

12. **Buy a puzzle book.** Make sure the book contains lots of beginner-level puzzles like word-finding puzzles, crosswords and Sudoku.

13. **Ask your loved one to help your children with their homework.** This is especially effective if the assignment has to do with a time in history your loved one remembers.

14. **Make a special treat like cocoa, sugar cookies and a sliced apple.** If he or she is able, let your loved one help prepare the treat. Enjoy it together and then let your loved one help you clean the kitchen and put everything away where it belongs.

15. **Make sure your loved one has books available.** If he or she can no longer read, read aloud. If your loved one does not appear to understand the words, use picture books.

16. **Ask your loved one to help you with a special project.** Ideas include sorting (blunt) tools and putting them away in your toolbox or untangling all of your costume jewelry.

17. **Buy or rent a DVD of your loved one's favorite television show or movie.** Watch the DVD as a family. Ask your loved one to explain why he or she likes the movie or television show so much.

18. **Help your loved one write a letter to a friend or a family member who lives out of town.** Allow him or her to send the letter through the mail.

19. **Sing some of your loved one's favorite songs together.** Don't correct him or her if they don't get all of the lyrics quite right.

20. **Look at old family photographs.** Encourage your loved one to tell you stories about family members you don't remember well or never had a chance to meet.

21. **Ask your loved one to tell you about historical events he or she remembers.** Ask about poignant events like the Great Depression, World War II, the Cuban Missile Crisis, or the assassination of President Kennedy, assuming these events do not cause him or her to become emotionally upset.

22. **Learn a new method of exercise together.** Choose something low-impact like yoga or Tai-Chi. This will not only improve your loved one's mood, but it will also help improve balance and reduce the likelihood of falls.

23. **Get out some art supplies like crayons, construction paper, glue, blunt scissors and glitter.** Encourage your loved one to draw pictures or design birthday or holiday cards to send to friends and family. Put a tarp on the table to protect the surface. Don't help unless your loved one asks you to do so.

24. **Take your loved one out to his or her favorite restaurant.** It's better to plan a lunch time visit. If you go in the evening, there may be too many people and your loved one may be struggling with sundowning. Whenever you decide to go, understand that you may have to leave if your loved one becomes tired or over-stimulated.

25. **Just sit quietly and hold your loved one's hand.** Simply being there can improve the health and happiness of your loved one.

Now that you've read our ideas, can you think of any other activities your loved one might enjoy? Don't be afraid to give them a try. If they work, that's great. If they don't, you can simply move on to something else.

CHAPTER FOURTEEN:
THE MANY FACETS OF PROVIDING CARE

Up until this point, we've focused on ways to improve the quality of your loved one's life; this chapter will address how you can best manage your own health and wellness while taking on this new responsibility. We have included this chapter specifically to help you. After all, you deserve it!

In these pages, you'll find information about several different types of caregiving, including long-distance caregiving, providing care to a loved one in your home, and how your role may change if your loved one moves to an assisted living or nursing facility. We will also discuss family dynamics that tend to be prominent when a parent needs care from adult children or when one spouse needs care from another. Finally, we will suggest several ways to manage stress and burnout.

Long-Distance Caregiving

Although Michelle loved her mother dearly, they both lived busy lives, Michelle in El Paso, Texas and her mother, Antonia, in a gated community in Miami. Sometimes they went weeks without speaking on the phone. Michelle had noticed over the past year that Antonia hadn't been very talkative during their infrequent calls, but she thought nothing of it. One night in July, Michelle was stunned to receive a phone call from a neighbor of Antonia's. Apparently, Antonia was living in squalor and had taken to roaming around the neighborhood in a nightgown. Michelle immediately traveled to Florida and took her mother to a doctor. The verdict was early- to middle-stage dementia. Now Michelle had some choices to make...

Like Michelle, out-of-town relatives may not be aware of the extent of their loved one's impairment. Even if you have phone contact regularly, the changes that come with the early stages of the disease may not be evident over the phone. Often, like Michelle, you will not have a true picture of your loved one's deficits until you get a call from one of his or her neighbors, friends, relatives that live close by, or more frighteningly, from the police or an adult protective services worker.

Once you are aware of your loved one's illness, you have three basic options. The first is to move your loved one into your home or into a facility near where you live. This allows you to manage his or her care without uprooting your life or the lives of others, such as your spouse and children. One problem with this decision is that it may remove your loved one from his or her support network. Antonia, for instance, had lived in Miami for more than 25 years. All of her friends were there. Uprooting her from the familiarity of home, friends, and neighbors could have a negative impact on her mental and emotional well-being, which could in turn lead to a decline in physical health.

Another option is to move to your loved one's town. Although this preserves your loved one's stability, it can mean a major upheaval in your life. Michelle was married with three school-aged children. She couldn't imagine relocating the whole family.

The final choice is to become a long-distance caregiver—to monitor your loved one's condition and care from hundreds of miles away. This is the choice Michelle made.

When you become a long-distance caregiver, you'll have to determine whether your loved one wants to remain at home with the support of a professional caregiver or whether he or she would prefer to be in a nursing facility. If you can afford to provide your loved one with 24/7 professional care in the home, this would benefit your loved one by eliminating the challenge of having to get used to a new living environment and the potential deterioration in emotional, physical and cognitive health that comes along with such an adjustment.

Being a long-distance caregiver has its challenges. You may get contradictory information from different healthcare professionals, your loved one's neighbors and other family members. Without being there to see things for yourself, it can be hard to figure out which information is "correct."

You will probably need to schedule visits to see your loved one on a regular basis so that you can make sure all is well. Additionally, you will want to set aside time and money for emergency trips if your loved one's condition declines significantly.

That said, long-distance caregiving can work well for both the caregiver and the patient. It may also be the most comfortable option, especially if your loved one has deep roots in his or her community.

In-Town Caregiving

Don felt his stomach knot as his cell phone rang...again. His father, Kevin, who lived alone and had been diagnosed with early-stage dementia, was calling Don for the tenth time that morning. This time it was to remind Don to bring milk when he stopped by for his evening visit. "I will, Dad," Don said, resisting the urge to add, "You've already told me that nine times!"

Whether your loved one lives at home or in a facility, one of the hardest things about being an in-town caregiver is that you are always at your loved one's beck and call—or you may feel you have to be. Since your loved one with dementia may forget that he or she has already called you once about an issue, you may get dozens of phone calls about the same thing. Facilities can handle this problem by restricting the resident's phone access, but if your loved one lives at home, you're fair game.

Though it can be stressful, there are pros to in-town caregiving: you can directly assess the changes in you loved one's condition without having to rely on the reports of others. Furthermore, it's easier to meet your loved one's needs on your own than it is to spend half a morning making phone calls to find someone several hundred miles away who will bring your loved one a gallon of milk.

Ironically, in-town caregivers often struggle more with guilt than long-distance caregivers. They often feel that, since their loved one has a life-limiting illness and lives so close by, they should be spending all their free time with him or her. Hiring a caregiver to visit two or three times per week to socialize with your loved one and run errands can remove some of the guilt: you gain peace of mind knowing your loved one's needs are being met by a compassionate, conscientious professional caregiver.

If your loved one calls constantly, it may be helpful to use reality orientation (see Chapter 10) by hanging a large calendar on your loved one's door. Fill in each day of the week with the name of the person who will be visiting and what he or she will do. For instance:

MONDAY – PAT (HOME CARE ASSISTANCE) 10AM – ERRANDS, PREPARING LUNCH AND LAUNDRY

WEDNESDAY – DON (SON) 6PM – ERRANDS AND DINNER OUT

FRIDAY – PAT (HOME CARE ASSISTANCE) 10AM – HELP WITH BATHING, PREPARING LUNCH, WALK TO THE PARK AND BACK

SUNDAY – DON (SON) 12PM – WATCH FOOTBALL AND PLAY CARD GAMES

In-Home Caregiving

Bringing your loved one into your home to provide care is a life-changing option for both you and your loved one. Before you take on the responsibility, talk to anyone that has worked with your loved one to get a clear picture of how much assistance he or she needs. Providing care for a loved one for an extended period of time can place a strain on family relationships, so it's also a good idea to talk to your spouse and children and get them on board before making the final decision.

You will also want to think about your own limits. Will you be comfortable giving your loved one a bath? Cleaning him or her up after an "accident?" If not, you may want to hire a caregiver to help handle your loved one's ADLs while you take care of the IADLs. (See Chapter Eleven for an explanation of these terms.) Finally, decide in advance if there will come a time when you will no longer be able to handle your loved one's care at home. Examples include:

- When she can no longer walk
- When he becomes incontinent
- When she starts to wander
- If he becomes sexually inappropriate or aggressive
- When she is bedbound
- When he is nearing the end of life and receiving hospice care

Write this limit down on a 3" x 5" index card and keep it in a place where you can see it every day. Although your boundaries may change as you become used to the tasks that caregiving requires, when you reach your limit and are near burnout, sit down with your family and discuss whether you want to continue to manage your loved one's care at home or whether it is time for him or her to receive care from a professional caregiver or to move to a nursing facility.

Caregiving When Your Loved One is in a Facility

Placing your loved one in a facility does not mean that your role as a caregiver is over, but it will change significantly. The facility will now be responsible for assisting with your loved one's ADLs. You, meanwhile, will have the chance to step back and relate to your loved one as a son, daughter, spouse, or friend. Try to visit and enjoy this relationship a few times each week, but don't necessarily feel like you have to make an appearance every day.

You will also team with the staff at the facility to make the best decisions regarding your loved one's care. Generally, within two weeks after admission, every three months thereafter, and whenever your loved one's condition changes significantly, the nursing facility will hold care plan meetings. These meetings are attended by nursing staff, social services staff, activities staff, dietary staff, and rehabilitative staff, if your loved one is receiving rehabilitation. Each professional gives a brief summary of your loved one's condition. You are then encouraged to share your observations and concerns, as well as ask any questions. Make an effort to attend every care plan meeting. If you can't be there physically, the care plan team can usually arrange to hold a phone conference with you. Some facilities also use Skype.

Much like in-town caregivers, caregivers whose loved ones have been placed in a nursing home may experience guilt. Doug Manning, author of When Love Gets Tough, a book that examines the dynamics of nursing home care, has observed that if a caregiver feels guilty about making the decision to place a loved one in a nursing facility, the facility will probably never satisfy his or her standards.

While you certainly have every right to expect that your loved one will receive compassionate, capable attention, you also have to realize that no nursing facility can provide the one-on-one care that your loved one would receive in a home care setting. He or she will occasionally be served a meal that is overcooked or not seasoned to taste and may not be continuously stimulated throughout the day. By all means, bring these matters to the attention of the staff, but don't let minutiae ruin your relationship with the nursing facility.

If you believe the facility is not taking good care of your loved one or if you believe your loved one is suffering abuse or neglect, notify the state and make arrangements to transfer your loved one to another facility.

Most people place their loved ones in a nursing facility expecting that the facility will be their final "home." As you will learn in Chapter Fifteen, "Dementia and End-of-Life Issues," people who are dying go through predictable declines including weight loss, an increased number of infections, withdrawal from others, declines in mobility and increased susceptibility to bed sores. It's important to remember that these declines would occur regardless of where your loved one lived and are out of the facility's control.

Family Dynamics

Families react in different ways to providing care to a loved one with dementia. The experience may bring a family closer together or cause irreparable damage.

Adult Children

In one of his recorded lectures, Doug Manning suggests that the adult child who ends up as the primary caregiver for one or both parents is often the "unblessed child," the child who never felt pretty enough or smart enough or good enough and who was never quite certain of his or her parents' love. As a result of these feelings, the child, now an adult, is often willing to bend over backwards to meet his or her parents' every need. All too often, he or she finds that, due to the dementia or to past family dynamics, he or she cannot please them. Meanwhile, the other siblings stay on the sidelines offering advice but no real assistance.

The only way to break free of this dynamic is for the unblessed child to find his or her voice and start setting clear, reasonable boundaries. "No, Mom, I can't come over to drive you to the grocery store right now. It's 3AM." "Jeff, I can't handle Mom every single day. I need you to go over to Mom's house and help her out at least three days a week. If you don't have the time, then please contribute the money so I can hire a professional caregiver."

On the other hand, some adult siblings become closer and mend broken bridges as they work to provide their loved one with the highest standards of care.

Gabe, Joe, and Melissa had very different personalities and had never been close, either as children or adults. When their 86-year-old mother, Wanda, began experiencing dementia symptoms, they started communicating, first by email, then by phone. Since none of the children lived in Chicago where Wanda did, they decided to hire a full-time home caregiver for her—each chipped in a third of the expense. Melissa, a nurse, said she'd stay in touch with their mother's doctors and make sure to let the home caregiver know about any medical appointments. Joe, a financial planner, said he'd take over managing their mother's money. They agreed he would send Gabe and Melissa a statement every quarter. Gabe, a minister and a social worker, said he would be sure Wanda continued to receive support from her church family and that he would be the primary contact for the home caregiver. The system worked beautifully, and even after Wanda passed away, Gabe, Joe, and Melissa retained their closeness.

If you want your family to draw closer together instead of slide further apart, you need to communicate clearly with each other. If you feel over-burdened, or if there is a job you're willing to assume, let your siblings know. Arrange to talk on the phone or communicate by email at least a few times a month. Try to spend some of that time focusing on the positives, such as the ways you are helping make your loved one's life better, instead of the negatives, such as how much stress is involved in caregiving.

Grandchildren

Young grandchildren may not remember their grandparent as he or she was before developing dementia. Older grandchildren, however, may have formed a relationship with their grandparent before the dementia developed. They may not understand why grandma can't remember their name anymore or why grandpa doesn't recall jokes that the two of them shared.

There are many excellent books for children about dementia (see Appendix A on Suggested Reading) that can help them understand their grandparent's condition. Many chapters of the Alzheimer's Association or the Alzheimer Society have support groups where children can share their questions and meet other kids their age who have a loved one with dementia.

If your loved one has withdrawn from other people or lashes out verbally, younger grandchildren may actually be afraid of him or her or think that they have done something to make him or her stop loving them. Explain to your children in language they can understand that their grandfather has a sickness in his brain that makes him forget things and that sometimes makes him angry. Be sure the grandchildren know that Grandpa's bad mood is not their fault.

Chances are good that if you are calm around your loved one with dementia, your children will soon feel at ease with him or her, too. Don't feel like you have to keep your loved one hidden away from your children. In fact, unless your loved one's behavior is physically or sexually aggressive, encourage your children to spend time around him or her. They will benefit from learning how to communicate with gentleness and respect; your loved one will benefit from the increased socialization. Communicating with grandchildren may even help stimulate your loved one's memory as he or she thinks back to share stories from his own childhood.

Spouses

People often make the assumption that caring for a spouse is easier than caring for a parent. After all, spouses are already intimately familiar with each other. There should be no cause for embarrassment as there might be between, say, a father and daughter or a mother and son.

Nevertheless, it is a difficult thing to go from viewing one's spouse as a life partner to viewing her as a cognitively impaired person in need of supervision and physical assistance. A caregiver spouse not only has to take over the huge amount of responsibility assumed by any other caregiver, he or she must do so while grieving the loss of a person he or she may think of as his or her closest friend. This is not to discount the grief felt by an adult child, who also may view her parent as a friend, but most spouses have had the unique experiences of meeting, falling in love and developing a partnership that has become the strongest part of their support system. To lose that support while, at the same time, assuming the job of caregiving can be a terrible and often unacknowledged loss.

Some spouses also have trouble setting limits on their loved one's behavior. This is especially true for women caring for their husbands. Older women are more likely to have been raised to listen to their husbands' decisions, not direct them as to what to do.

Jennifer frequently allowed her husband, Stan, to wander outside at night. He inevitably became lost. After returning Stan to his home several times, a police officer asked Jennifer why on earth she let Stan go out at night. Jennifer gave the officer a horrified look. "Oh," she said, "it's not my place to tell my husband what to do!"

If you find yourself having trouble changing roles from lover to caregiver, you are not alone. It may help to go to a support group for spouses and partners of people with dementia. You can find one through the Alzheimer's Association or the Alzheimer Society.

It's also important to stay in touch with your friends and accept support from them. Some of your friends may be reluctant to call because they don't know what to say to you. Take the initiative and call them. Let them know how your spouse is doing and how they can help. It's also important to ask for and accept help from your adult children.

Caregiver Stress Relievers

We all relieve stress in different ways. You may find comfort in taking a hike, going dancing with friends, or simply having some time to relax alone and read a few chapters of your favorite book. In other words, all the ideas presented here won't work for every single person. Use the ones that help, ignore the ones that don't, and don't be afraid to think up relaxing plans on your own. Some relaxation techniques that many caregivers have found useful include:

- Eating a healthy diet (but comfort foods are okay, too!).
- Limiting alcohol and steer clear of recreational drugs.
- Doing something physical at least three times a week.
- Talking to supportive friends and family members as often as possible.
- Going out with friends at least once a week. Don't talk about dementia.
- Getting a massage.
- Joining a support group.

- Going for a drive in your car. (Scream if you feel like it.)
- Reading your favorite book.
- Going to your church, synagogue, or mosque.
- Going to a movie.
- Getting away for the weekend.
- Watching a movie that makes you laugh out loud.
- Watching a movie that makes you cry.
- Writing all your thoughts down in a journal.
- Adopting a pet from a homeless shelter and spending time petting and playing with it.
- Looking in the mirror every morning and saying, "I know I can do this."

CHAPTER FIFTEEN:
DEMENTIA AND END-OF-LIFE ISSUES

Progressive dementia is considered a terminal condition. Depending on the type of dementia from which your loved one suffers, the course of the disease may be as short as just a few years or as long as 20 years.

No matter what the course, loss is always significant and can be stressful, especially if you are called upon to make emergency medical decisions on your loved one's behalf.

This chapter will discuss some of the most common causes of death among people with dementia. It will also take a look at some of the decisions you may be asked to make and what implications those decisions may have for your loved one. Finally, we will introduce the concept of hospice care and how it can improve your loved one's comfort level.

Common Causes of Death

Many people do not realize that dementia itself can be a cause of death. Alzheimer's disease, for example, is the fifth leading cause of death among people over the age of 65 years. The mechanism is not completely understood, but most researchers believe that, as the brain suffers more and more damage, the structures that regulate life functions such as breathing, swallowing, and maintaining a regular heart rhythm start to fail. In the end, the brain simply cannot sustain life.

Another common cause of death among dementia patients is pneumonia, usually caused by aspiration. Aspiration occurs when the brain can no longer regulate swallowing. As a result, the person may inhale food into the lungs when he or she tries to eat. The food is recognized as a foreign body and causes an infection—pneumonia—to develop in the lungs.

Heart disease is another common cause of death among individuals with dementia. The relationship between heart disease and vascular dementia is relatively straightforward, as both involve blood flow problems. Research has also revealed, however, that people with cardiovascular problems have an increased risk for developing Alzheimer's disease; the relationship between these conditions remains unclear. In any case, both heart disease and dementia, whether vascular or Alzheimer's disease, are more common with increasing age. People with vascular dementia are also likely to experience strokes, which is another common cause of death.

Hard Choices

If you are going to make health care choices for your loved one, you will need to be listed as your loved one's agent on his DPOA for health care. You may also be guided by a "Do Not Resuscitate" order or a living will (all these documents are explained in Chapter Five).

The first thing you will need to decide is whether you want your loved one to receive aggressive (curative) treatment at a hospital or to be kept comfortable at a home or in a nursing facility with palliative (comfort) care. Keep in mind that hospitalization might cure the current problem, such as pneumonia, but it will not stop the dementia process or prevent death from happening eventually.

If your loved one goes to the hospital, the next decision you will have to make involves whether or not to place him or her on a ventilator, or breathing machine. Ventilators were not intended to help severely damaged lungs, and they may or may not prolong your loved one's life.

Finally, you will be asked if you want your loved one to receive nutrition through a feeding tube, which is surgically implanted in the stomach. Again, the feeding tube may provide nutrition for a short time, but it will not cure the dementia.

The Alzheimer's Association has stated in their publications, "The evidence and research suggest that all efforts at life extension in the advanced stages of Alzheimer's creates burdens and avoidable suffering for patients who could otherwise live out the remainder of their lives in greater comfort and peace." Of course any decisions are left to the discretion of you and the wishes your loved one may have prepared in advance.

Hospice Care

Hospice is a program that is covered by Medicare, Medicaid, and most types of private insurance. It is designed to provide comfort care to people who have been given a prognosis of six months or less to live. Hospice can work with your loved one wherever he or she lives—at home, at an assisted living facility or at a skilled nursing facility.

Hospice teams are managed by a nurse, who works with you to accomplish your loved one's care. Other team members include a social worker, a home health aide to help with personal care, a chaplain, and a volunteer coordinator.

Hospice workers are skilled at identifying and relieving symptoms of discomfort. They typically avoid any measures that could be painful to your loved one, such as shots, IVs, and other invasive procedures.

Hospice attends not only to the needs of the patient, they also provide education and support for family members. When the patient dies, the hospice nurse visits to assist the family with contacting the funeral home of their choice. Afterwards, hospice remains available to family members and friends to provide bereavement counseling.

If your loved one is in late-stage dementia and you do not want him or her to receive any curative treatment, hospice is a good option to care for your loved one and offer understanding and support to you.

CONCLUSION

Dementia has been called "the long goodbye" because it steals our loved ones from us a bit at a time . . . a memory here . . . a forgotten name there . . . a misplaced purse . . . a blank look at the once-beloved face of a spouse, a child, or a grandchild.

Through much of the early stage of dementia, physical care isn't even required. As a caregiver, your job is to provide supervision, making sure the environment is as safe as possible, and support cognitive stimulation with activities, games, coaching, cues, and instruction.

It can feel like a futile battle, because in the end, you never know for sure how much you have improved your loved one's quality of life or how many coherent moments you've won.

The time you spend with your loved one, however, is not futile. Not the memory games you play to help increase concentration and focus, nor the hours you spend reading aloud when he or she can no longer read because of brain damage, nor the days you spend holding the hand of a loved one who hasn't spoken to you or recognized you in more than a year.

Here at Home Care Assistance, we recognize that all of your time with your loved one is important, and we want to help you make that time as meaningful as possible. Our Balanced Care Method™ is designed to provide unparalleled levels of care and companionship to our clients. Let us focus on meeting his or her physical needs so that you can focus on being a family member.

And if dementia is your loved one's challenge, we hope you'll consider taking advantage of our Dementia Therapeutics™ program. Based on years of research, we provide specially trained interventionists, coaches and care specialists to help your loved one maintain her highest level of cognitive functioning and quality of life that is possible.

If we can in any way help to make your job as a dementia caregiver easier, please contact us online at **http://www.HomeCareAssistance.com** or by phone at **1-866-454-8346**.

APPENDIX A:
SUGGESTED READINGS

The 36-Hour Day: A Family Guide to Caring for People Who Have Alzheimer Disease, Related Dementias, and Memory Loss (5th Edition), by Nancy L. Mace and Peter V. Rabins (The Johns Hopkins University Press, 2011).

The Alzheimer's Legal Survival Guide, by William G. Hammond, Karen Hays Weber, Mary Helen Gautreaux, and Mary-Lane Kamberg (The Elder & Disability Law Firm, 2000).

American Medical Association Guide to Home Caregiving, by the American Medical Association (Wiley, 2001).

A Caregiver's Guide to Alzheimer's Disease: 300 Tips for Making Life Easier, by Patricia Callone, Barbara Vasiloff, Roger Brumback, Janaan Manternach, and Connie Kudlacek (Demos Medical Publishing, 2005).

A Caregiver's Guide to Lewy Body Dementia, by Helen Buell Whitworth and Jim Whitworth (Demos Health, 2010).

The Complete Eldercare Planner, Revised and Updated Edition: Where to Start, Which Questions to Ask, and How to Find Help, by Joy Loverde (Three Rivers Press, 2009).

A Dignified Life: The Best Friends Approach to Alzheimer's Care, A Guide for Family Caregivers, by Virginia Bell and David Troxel (HCI, 2002).

Elder Rage or Take My Father, Please!: How to Survive Caring for Aging Parents, by Jacqueline Marcell (Impressive Press, 2001).

Eldercare for Dummies, by Rachelle Zukerman (For Dummies, 2003).

The Emotional Survival Guide for Caregivers: Looking after Yourself and Your Family While Helping an Aging Parent, by Barry J. Jacobs (The Guilford Press, 2006).

From Hospital to Home Care: A Step by Step Guide to Providing Care to Patients Post Hospitalization, by Kathy N. Johnson, James H. Johnson, and Lily Sarafan (Home Care Press, 2012).

The Good Caregiver: A One-of-a-Kind Compassionate Resource for Anyone Caring for Aging Loved Ones, by Robert L. Kane (Avery Trade, 2011).

Gone from My Sight: The Dying Experience by Barbara Karnes (Barbara Karnes Books, 2008).

The Handbook of Live in Care: A Guide for Caregivers, by Kathy N. Johnson, James H. Johnson, and Lily Sarafan (Home Care Press, 2011).

Hard Choices for Loving People: CPR, Artificial Feeding, Comfort Care and the Patient with a Life Threatening Illness, 5th Edition by Hank Dunn (A & A Publishers, 2009).

How You Can Survive When They're Depressed: Living and Coping with Depression Fallout, by Anne Sheffield (Three Rivers Press, 1999).

Keeping Busy: A Handbook of Activities for Persons with Dementia, by James R. Dowling (The Johns Hopkins University Press, 1995).

Loving Someone Who Has Dementia: How to Find Hope While Coping with Stress and Grief, by Pauline Boss (Jossey-Bass, 2011).

Making the Moments Count: Leisure Activities for Caregiving Relationships, by Joanne Ardolf Decker (The Johns Hopkins University Press, 1997).

Striped Shirts and Flowered Pants: A Story about Alzheimer's Disease for Young Children, by Barbara Schnurbush (Magination Press, 2007).

Talking to Alzheimer's: Simple Ways to Connect When You Visit with a Family Member or Friend, by Claudia J. Strauss (New Harbinger Publications, 2002).

What's Happening to Grandpa? By Maria Shriver (Little, Brown Books for Young Readers, 2004).

When Love Gets Tough: The Nursing Home Decision by Doug Manning (In Sight Books, 2006).

APPENDIX B:

WEB-BASED RESOURCES FOR SENIORS AND/OR CAREGIVERS

AARP - http://www.aarp.org/
Provides political advocacy, discounts, and information to senior citizens.

Agency for Healthcare Research and Quality -
http://www.ahrq.gov/research/elderix.htm
Reviews the results of evidence-based healthcare studies about seniors.

Alzheimer Society - http://www.alzheimer.ca/
Alzheimer's information and support in Canada

Alzheimer's Association - http://www.alz.org/
Funds research and provides information and support to families dealing with Alzheimer's.

Canadian Caregiver Coalition - http://www.ccc-ccan.ca/
Provides advocacy, leadership, research, education, information, communication and resources development to caregivers in Canada.

Canadian Centre for Elder Law - http://www.bcli.org/ccel
Conducts research, outreach, and education on elder law issues in Canada.

Canadian Dementia Action Network - http://www.cdan.ca/
Dedicated to finding a cure as well as helping those currently living with dementia and their families.

Canadian Senior Years - http://www.senioryears.com/
Information, articles, news, links, email pal service.

Home Care Assistance - http://www.homecareassistance.com
Provides non-medical home-based health care to seniors.

Medicare.org - http://www.alz.org/
Provides information about and assistance accessing the government-backed health insurance plan which covers most seniors in the United States.

Seniors Canada Online -
http://www.seniors.gc.ca/h.4m.2@.jsp?lang=eng
Information and services for Canadian seniors.

National Family Caregiver's Association -
http://www.nfcacares.org/index.cfm
US-based site offering education, support, empowerment and advocacy to caregivers.

National Institute on Aging - http://www.nia.nih.gov/
Conducts geriatric research and provides information to seniors and their families.

Nifty after Fifty - http://www.niftyafterfifty.com/
Fitness information for seniors.

Public Health Agency of Canada, Aging and Seniors -
http://www.phac-aspc.gc.ca/seniors-aines/index-eng.php
Provides medical information for Canadian Seniors

USA.gov., Senior Citizens' Resources -
http://www.usa.gov/Topics/Seniors.shtml
List of links to other resources dealing with health care, caregiver resources, and end of life issues.

OUR MISSION

Our mission at Home Care Assistance is to change the way the world ages. We provide older adults with quality care that enables them to live happier, healthier lives at home. Our services are distinguished by the caliber of our caregivers, the responsiveness of our staff and our expertise in Live-In care. We embrace a positive, balanced approach to aging centered on the evolving needs of older adults.

- Live-In Experts. We specialize in around the clock care to help seniors live well at home.

- Available 24/7. Care managers are on call for clients and their families, even during nights and weekends.

- High Caliber Caregivers. We hire only 1 in 25 applicants and provide ongoing training and supervision.

- Balanced Care. Our unique approach to care promotes healthy mind, body and spirit.

- No Long Term Contracts. Use our services only as long as you're 100% satisfied.

- A Trusted Partner. We're honored to be Preferred Providers for professionals in both the medical and senior communities.

- Peace of Mind. Independent industry surveys place our client satisfaction rate at 97%.

AUTHOR BIOGRAPHIES

Samuel T. Gontkovsky, PsyD is a neuropsychologist and Director of Dementia Therapeutics. He has more than 15 years of experience in clinical practice, research, teaching, and administration. He holds a doctorate in Clinical Psychology from Nova Southeastern University.

Kathy N. Johnson, PhD, CMC is a Certified Geriatric Care Manager serving the San Francisco Bay Area. She holds a Doctorate in Psychology from the Illinois Institute of Technology.

James H. Johnson, PhD is a licensed clinical psychologist and the award-winning author of seven books. A former university professor and department chair, he holds a Doctorate in Psychology from the University of Minnesota.

Lily Sarafan, MS is a corporate executive and advocate in the senior care industry. She holds Masters and Bachelors degrees from Stanford University.

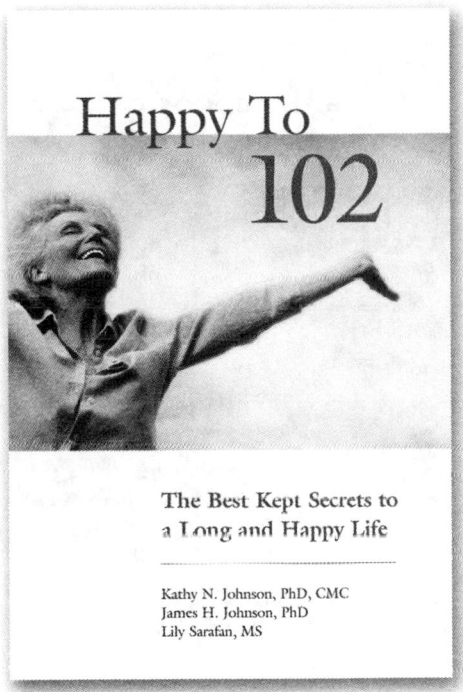

Available on **amazon**.com.

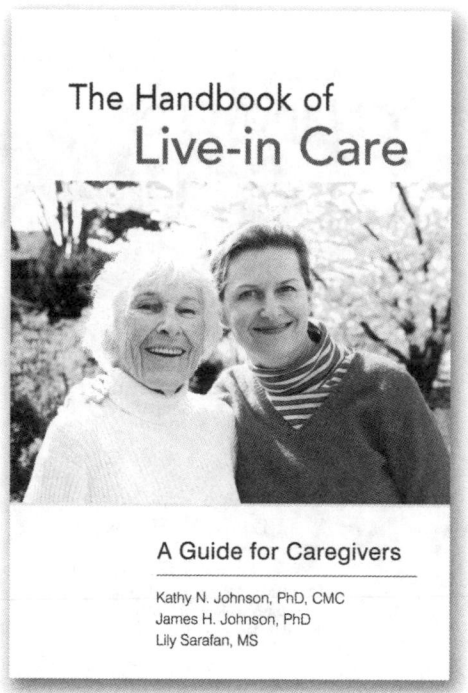

Available on **amazon**.com.

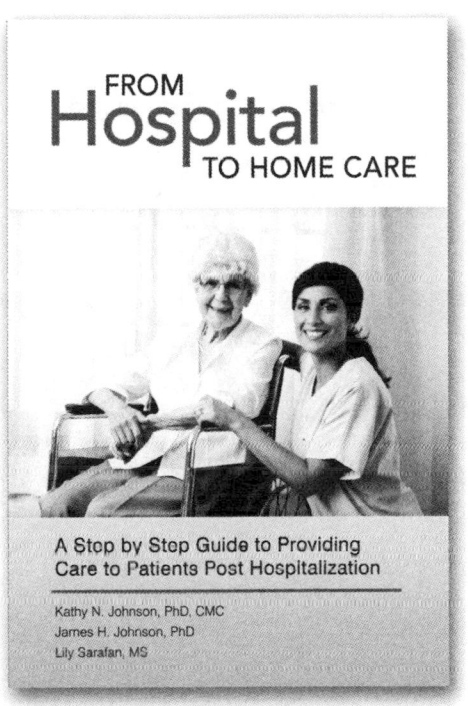

Available on **amazon**.com.

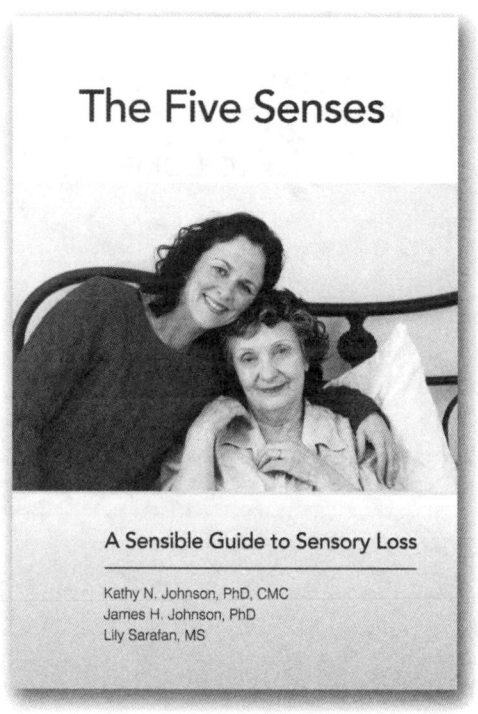

NOTES

NOTES

NOTES

NOTES

NOTES

NOTES

NOTES

NOTES

NOTES

NOTES